CHRONIC

BACK PAIN:

MOVING ON

Julie Zimmerman, PT

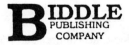

BIDDLE
PUBLISHING
COMPANY

PO Box 1305 #103, Brunswick, Maine 04011

Copyright © 1991

by

Biddle Publishing Company

Publisher's Cataloging in Publication Data
1 - Zimmerman, Julie
2 - Chronic Back Pain: Moving On
3 - Bibliography, Appendix C
   Includes Index
4 - Backache
   Chronic pain
   Health, back care
   Medical self - care
   Medical treatment of chronic back pain
   Self - care, health
   Treatment of chronic back pain
Library of Congress Catalog Card Number 90 - 85648
ISBN 1 - 879418 - 04 - 5

Dedication

To Susan, Lloyd and all the other health professionals who join their chronic pain patients in the search for answers

and

To Sandy, Barbara and all the other friends and family members who respect the decision to end the search

Chronic Back Pain

It begins with the fear
   of missing another meeting, another party, breaking another promise;
   soon afraid of
   losing a career? a future?
   becoming a burden, a bore
   every move necessitating the question – Will this make me worse?
   "I can't." at home, at work
   "Don't count on me."

   What can I count on?

The guilt
   the responsible one no longer fulfilling the responsibilities – others doing
my share, pulling my weight,
   or – it's not done
   the dust on the floor soon becomes incidental
   the commitments unhonored continue to gnaw

The frustration
   not constant, flaring up in bursts of resentment –
   with a new standard of activity, the mind shuts off all I used to do
   until, shattering acceptance,
"I can never do that again!"
   I crave spontaneity, to stop being careful

   Old before I enter middle age

Self-esteem, badly shaken
   independence and accomplishment no longer automatic
   I was contributing, productive, busy –
What am I now?
   after accepting the prognosis, trying hard to learn the new life-style,
regain a sense of myself
   confidence threatened by every piece of advice from well-meaning friends
on what I should be trying

1

anxious to leave behind the desperate hope for an instant cure
and get on with my life

Secondary to these, the pain
  the chief symptom,
  the guide for the future
  not insupportable at any one moment, though draining and demoralizing
over time
  but important mostly in the limitations it dictates

  almost a relief when the doctors agree – "learn to live with it"
  time to accept the pain, to make the changes that will control it

And, surprisingly, the compensations
  the concern and expressions of love from friends –
the gift of their time and effort
  the assurance from my husband – I'm still his choice, despite my losses
  a new awareness of self, a new perspective on life
  discovering new pleasures, new goals, reserves of strength
  to learn that my value is not in what I can do,
  but in what I am

An object of compassion?
still compassionate
still glad to be me

Julie Zimmerman

Chronic Back Pain: Moving On

Table of Contents

Author's Preface

When I began the search to find a cure for the debilitating back pain that was disrupting my life, I visited my family doctor, an orthopedic surgeon, a neurologist, a neurosurgeon, a rheumatologist, two osteopaths, an acupuncturist and two physical therapists. I tried a corset, acupuncture and the acupuncture diet, manipulation, various medications, bedrest, ultrasound, massage therapy, exercise programs, posture training, foot orthotics and positive thinking. I was advised to base my activity level on the pain and advised to ignore the pain. I was told that I should turn the pain over to God, that I should let myself get well and that my physical problem was a direct result of spiritual negativity. Friends insisted that osteopathy is the one answer, that acupuncture is the one answer and that chiropractic is the one answer. Diagnoses considered included muscle strain, degenerative disk disease, lupus (SLE), rheumatoid arthritis, somatic dysfunction, multiple sclerosis, prolapsed disks, piriformis syndrome and sacro-iliac joint dysfunction. My official diagnosis remains "low back pain".

One of the brightest days in the months of medical appointments and trial treatment was the day my family doctor, husband and I had a conference; we decided that the search for a diagnosis and cure had gone on long enough, that I have a disability which is probably permanent and that it was finally time to get on with my life. It was distressing to give up my career as a physical therapist, a vocation that had absorbed and defined me for years, but it was also an enormous relief to let go of the commitments I could no longer honor.

Chronic pain is with me daily, straining my physical and emotional resources. There is a struggle to maintain self-esteem, but also the emergence of new interests and new horizons. My back pain hasn't diminished in the years since its onset, but I consider myself to be a happy, productive person; it was impossible to be either when my only goal was to resume my former pain-free life. Now I can say "I'm fine!" and mean it.

While searching for answers to my own condition and in my professional research and experience, I have learned how controversial and complicated back pain is. My hope is that *Chronic Back Pain: Moving On* can help those of you with chronic or recurrent back pain find the ways to minimize your pain and proceed with your lives.

Introduction: Misdiagnoses and Unsuccessful Treatments

"We are spending too much on treatments that are not proven and on diseases that aren't actually there." Charles Federspiel, PhD[6]

200 million of 250 million Americans will have back trouble before age 50;[1] in people younger than 45 it is the most frequent cause of disability. Back pain is the nation's most common musculoskeletal complaint, with 7 million disabled annually.[25] For 10 percent, or 20 million, the symptoms will become chronic. Back pain, the most expensive benign condition in America, costs up to $80 billion/year in lost wages and productivity,[2] plus many billions more in medical costs, disability claims, lawsuits and related expenses; no other affliction even comes close. Back problems are second only to upper respiratory infections for causing missed work and visits to the family doctor; they are responsible for the largest number of workers' compensation claims and up to 32 percent of disability payments.[25]

The phenomenal scope of this problem should mean that it is well understood. Unfortunately, the controversy surrounding the diagnosis and treatment of back pain proves otherwise. People with back pain frequently receive a variety of diagnoses, misdiagnoses or no diagnosis; finding the right treatment is often a matter of luck. Back pain may continue for months or years despite patients' best efforts and those of their heath care providers.

Diagnosis

"Early, accurate diagnosis is not absolutely essential." Mark Horwich, M.D.[16]
"The cause of chronic pain is a lack of diagnosis; truly effective, relieving treatment is unlikely without a diagnosis." William Wyatt, D.O. [34]

A patient who consults a GP, chiropractor, orthopedic surgeon, osteopath and alternative healer may get five different opinions as to the cause of his back pain. Each health practitioner seems to have a different explanation for a patient's symptoms. Many patients never receive a specific diagnosis and are classified as suffering from "low back syndrome".[31] The majority will never know the true underlying cause of their pain.[26] In fact, few back injuries can be traced to anatomical disorders and no medical test or examination technique can say what actually caused them.[22,30]

Although the principle obligation of a health care professional is to diagnose and treat pathology, there is often little to go on but the patient's report of pain. Health practitioners who treat back pain base treatment on their individualized views of what causes it and in which spinal structures the pain originates; the variation of opinions is staggering!

- *"Trauma is the most frequent cause of back pain, the main reason being that people are in poor physical condition."*[3]
- *"80 percent of back pain is caused by weak or tense muscles."*[33]
- *"50-70 percent of chronic symptoms are psychological in origin."*[5-A]
- *"The majority of lower-back pain actually originates in the sacral ligaments."*[8]
- *"An extremely high percentage of patients with pain have fascial problems."*[7]
- *"The majority of chronic disabling low back pain is from degenerative changes."*[17]
- *"Most neck, shoulder and back pain is due to Tension Myositis Syndrome."*[29]
- *"In 50 percent or more of back pain patients, the facet joint is the site of dysfunction."*[5-B]
- *"Chronic pain is caused by chronic guilt; back problems are due to a lack of feeling supported."*[15]
- *"Chronic sprain is probably the most common low back problem."*[21]
- *"Functional disorders of the musculoskeletal system called somatic dysfunctions are responsible for most (95 percent) back pain."*[4]
- *"90-95 percent of back pain is due to disks."*[5-C]
- *"Vertebral subluxations are found in every sick, malfunctioning body."*[20]
- *"Improper diet and lifestyle are the root of most of our medical problems."*[18]
- And from a British newspaper, *"There is a well-proven relationship between the number of cigarettes smoked and the likelihood the individual will have back problems."*

Introduction

Obviously, the health care profession does not have a firm grasp on the condition which affects 80 percent of Americans. This is frightening for the person with back pain who wants to know immediately and with certainty 'What's wrong?' 'How serious is it?,' 'Will it get worse?,' and 'What do I do?' Most people assume that curative treatment can't begin until a health problem is accurately diagnosed. In the field of back pain, it is commonplace for treatment to be prescribed without a diagnosis or with a misdiagnosis.

Treatment

"Researchers say there's no clear-cut advantage of one kind of treatment over another." David Zinman [35]

"The vast majority of approaches to treating back pain patients have been found to be no better than no treatment at all." James McGavin, PT [24]

Given the lack of agreement concerning the diagnosis of back pain, it is not surprising that treatment for the condition is equally controversial. Treatment is often based on the philosophy and training of the practitioner rather than the patient's symptoms. Regardless of the treatment approach, 60-80 percent recover from an acute low back pain episode in three days to three weeks;[9] 90 percent recover within two months.[10] Most back aches get better despite treatment rather than because of it. When spontaneous recovery and medical intervention fail, back pain becomes chronic. Treatment continues, but it is often expensive, inappropriate and prescribed in response to the patient's pain level, not to address known pathology. The desperate wish for a quick fix also encourages non-conventional approaches which may be harmful. Many patients shop around and try, in the words of one neurosurgeon, *"injections, stimulators, mechanical devices, and Rolfing, none of which can possibly have any curative effect."* [14]

Although an army of "experts" claims that they have found the answer for "most" back pain patients, this field has a dismal percentage of cure. Claims made concerning the success of various treatments cannot be taken at face value; if the following statements were all true, one would be at a loss to understand why so many Americans suffer from recurrent or chronic back pain.

- *"I haven't seen any techniques that are so effective in reducing pain and restoring function as myofascial release."* [7]

8

- *"Mobilization and manipulation studies claim an 80 percent success rate."* [11]

- *"80 percent of low back pain patients get immediate relief with epidural blocks."* [32]

- *"In one study, the McKenzie approach revealed that 97 percent of patients improved over one week of treatment."* [24]

- *"With Meridian Therapy 40 percent were still free of complaints after one year and 30 percent were better."* [12]

- *"With microcurrent therapy, 95 percent of patients got pain relief and 82 percent were pain free within 10 treatments."* [27]

- *"90 percent of patients diagnosed with sacroiliac joint dysfunction without secondary factors obtained significant relief with manipulation."* [24]

- *"Radiofrequency facet denervation is more than 70 percent effective."* [28]

- *"95 percent were better or cured with manipulation under anesthesia preceded by a full eclectic regimen."* [19]

- *"In the YMCA's exercise program, 80 percent improve and 31 percent have pain completely eliminated."* [33]

- *"70-80 percent of those carefully screened for radicular symptoms benefit from surgery."* [9]

Although every technique helps some people with back pain, nothing works for everyone. Practitioners who diagnose the same problem and prescribe the same treatment regime for every patient don't help the majority of their patients. The onus is often on the patient to believe in a treatment in order for it to work, implying that those without optimistic attitudes will undermine the healer's efforts. However, it is unfair to expect people searching for relief to get their hopes up again and again. Practitioners of a specific philosophy shouldn't demand total commitment from a patient, but rather an open mind. The test of a treatment's success is what works in the long run.

Fortunately, the people whose back pain signals a potentially serious disease have a good chance of being accurately diagnosed and effectively treated. The other 85-90 percent [6,13] are usually diagnosed with "low back syndrome" or with one of the conditions which falls into this category, (such as degenerative disk disease, muscle strain and sacro-iliac joint dysfunction). These syndromes can be extraordinarily painful and limiting, but are not life-threatening; there are many treatment and management options which can provide relief.

Introduction

Learn to Live With It

When back pain reaches the six-month milestone, people are suddenly and dramatically transformed into "CHRONIC PAIN PATIENTS." In the eyes of the health profession, the prognosis immediately deteriorates; family and friends may become less solicitous; the patient reaches the depths of discouragement. Society seems to admire those people who "tough it out," but it is impossible to keep functioning normally while ignoring a high level of pain which continues indefinitely. Toughing it out is emotionally exhausting; eventually one's disposition and coping mechanisms are strained to the limit.

The day finally comes when the patient is told "you have to learn to live with it." This statement is often thrown up as an example of uncaring, unfeeling doctors. However, learning to live with chronic pain is not necessarily losing the battle. After months spent in the search for a diagnosis or cure, it may come as a relief to be able to leave that whole process of waiting and disappointment behind, make the necessary adaptations and get on with life. Some believe that accepting a disability is giving up and that pain can be overcome with sufficient willpower. A positive attitude has an important role in health and recovery, but no one should be held responsible for continuing to have symptoms. There are many people with great determination who cannot reverse their pain and dysfunction with a fighting attitude. Instead they face the challenge by forging a meaningful life in spite of their disabilities.

People with back pain may never know for sure if their pain is curable. How many specialists and alternative approaches should they try? Are the time, money, waiting and risk of side effects worth it for each new attempt? How long do they look for a cure before making permanent changes in their lives? These questions have to be answered on an individual basis; they depend on level of disability, severity of symptoms, financial and time restraints. A general guideline is to listen to all the advice, research the treatment approaches, weigh the risks, get recommendations for specific practitioners and give the appropriate methods a fair try. After doing one's best, within reason, to find an effective treatment, it is then appropriate to accept the peace that comes with "learning to live with it".

Chronic Back Pain: Moving On gives individuals with back problems the knowledge to better understand the effects of chronic pain and the measures that can be taken to control it. What works to a patient's advantage is to be as informed as possible about backs and what can happen to them. PART 1 looks at the normal and dysfunctional back and at the differences between acute and chronic pain; it examines chronic pain from both the professional and personal points of view. PART 2 discusses the treatment options and their rationales for people with chronic back pain. Pain inhibition and pain management techniques, combined with a home treatment program and self-help adaptations, can allow people with this disability to maximize their physical and emotional resources and minimize their pain.

Using *Chronic Back Pain: Moving On*

1) The information presented in this book is based in part on the writings and research of practitioners in the field of back pain. Given the considerable controversy in this area, an attempt has been made to discuss opposing theories objectively and fairly.

2) In keeping with the attempt to present information objectively, the book is written in the third person. The exception is in sections which offer specific recommendations to "you," the person with back pain.

3) Certain sections provide in-depth or technical information on specific topics. These are boxed so that readers not interested in such detail can easily continue with the basic text.

4) For those unfamiliar with anatomical terms, the first chapter, "The Normal Back/The Painful Back," explains the anatomy and movement of the spine and the medical problems which can affect it. A complete glossary is included in Appendix A.

5) At the end of every chapter is a summary or overview of the information in that chapter, titled "Key Points."

6) Footnotes throughout the text refer to the numbered resources listed alphabetically at the end of each chapter. A complete bibliography is included in Appendix C.

7) People with acute back pain are "patients" during the diagnostic process and while receiving professional treatment. When a person's pain becomes chronic, the "patient" designation is no longer appropriate. In this book, people are referred to as "patients" only in the context of diagnosis and treatment.

8) *Chronic Back Pain: Moving On* is written for the person with back pain,

but is also appropriate for the health practitioner who treats back pain patients. Chronic pain is a frustrating condition to treat as well as to live with; patients and practitioners need to understand each other's point of view.

Disclaimer

The purpose of *Chronic Back Pain: Moving On* is to provide information regarding chronic back pain and its treatment and management options. It should be used as a general guide and readers should tailor all information to their individual circumstances. **This book is in no way meant to take the place of an individualized evaluation and treatment plan from a qualified health professional.**

The author and Biddle Publishing Company have neither liability nor responsibility to any person with respect to any injury alleged to be caused directly or indirectly by the information contained in this book. If the reader does not wish to be bound by the above, the book may be returned to the publisher for a full refund.

Footnotes

1 Edward Abraham, *Freedom from Back Pain*
2 Henry Allen, "That Back's Gotta Come Out"
3 American Medical Association, *Book of Back Care*
4 American Osteopathic Association, informational literature
5 "Approaches to Musculoskeletal Problems: Focus on the Low Back" Symposium, (A–Jane Derebery, B–Frederick Carrick, C–Robert Boyd)
6 *The Back Letter*, Vol. 4, No. 3
7 John Barnes, "Benefits of Myofascial Release, Craniosacral Therapy Explained"
8 Ben Benjamin, "The Mystery of Lower Back Pain"
9 Rene Cailliet, *Low Back Pain Syndrome*
10 Consumer Reports Books, *Health Quackery*
11 Richard DiFabio, "Clinical Assessment of Manipulation and Mobilization of the Lumbar Spine"
12 Jan Dommerholt, "Meridian Therapy – A New European Concept"
13 Richard DonTigny, "Function and Pathomechanics of the Sacroiliac Joint"
14 Charles Fager, "Facts and Fallacies of Spinal Disorders: A Neurosurgeon's View"
15 Louise Hay, *You Can Heal Your Life*
16 Mark Horwich, "Low Back Pain: The Neurologist's View"
17 Bernard Jacobs, "Low Back Pain: The Orthopedist's View"
18 Ronald Kotzch, "AIDS: Putting an Alternative to the Test"
19 Krumhansl & Nowacek, "Case Study – Spinal Manipulation Under Anaesthesia"

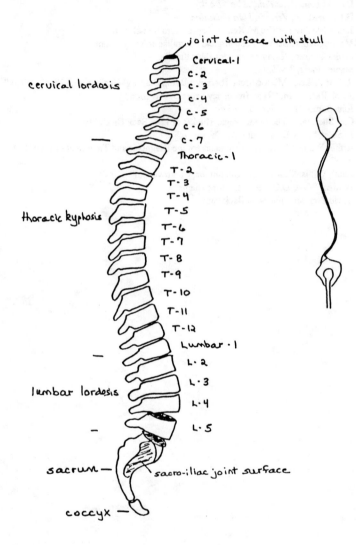

Figure 1-1. The spinal column, side view.

PART 1 - CHRONIC PAIN

Chapter 1 - The Normal Back/The Painful Back

Normal Anatomy of the Spine

"The thigh bone's connected to the hip bone, the hip bone's connected to the back bone, the back bone's connected to the neck bone, now hear the word of the Lord!" Source Unknown

"The back" functions as a single unit, but it is a complex structure composed of bones, joints, disks, muscles, ligaments, a spinal cord, nerve roots and all their connective and surrounding tissues. The back is shaped and supported by individual bony segments, the **vertebrae**; together they make up the vertebral or **spinal column**. The spinal column has four built-in curves, two concavities ("lordoses") of the low back and neck, and two convexities ("kyphoses") of the upper back and sacrum. These allow energy-efficient postural balance and serve a shock-absorbing role for the body. The spinal column is divided into five sections; the seven **cervical**, twelve **thoracic** and five **lumbar vertebrae** are separate bones, while the five **sacral vertebrae** are fused into one bone, the **sacrum**. The **coccyx**, or tailbone, is also one fused entity. [see Figure 1-1]

15

The spinal column is joined at the sacrum to the **pelvis**; this large bone is a ring composed of three sections (ilium, ischium and pubis). The sacro-iliac joints join the ilia of the pelvis to the sacrum; the pubic bones are connected anteriorly by strong fibrous tissue (the "pubic symphysis"). [see Figure 1-2]

Structures Joining Vertebra to Vertebra

(1) Intervertebral **disks** sit between the bodies of the vertebrae and provide cushioning and shock absorption; they have a tough fibrous outer ring (the "annulus fibrosis") and soft gelatin-like center (the "nucleus pul-posis"). [see Figures 1-3 & 1-5]

(2) Each vertebra has seven bony projections or prominences – a spinous process posteriorly, two transverse processes laterally and four articular proces-ses which extend up or down. [see Figures 1-4 & 1-5] **Facet joints** link the two superior articular processes of one vertebra to the two inferior articular processes of the vertebra above it. [see Figures 1-6 & 1-7] [see Box 1-1]

Facet Joints

Joints are interruptions in the skeleton where movement occurs; facet joints allow movement between the vertebrae. They are "synovial" type joints, as are most joints with detectable amounts of movement. Synovial joints are so-called because they are lined by a "synovial membrane" that produces fluid for lubrication and protection; a "joint capsule" surrounds and encloses the joint. Some synovial joints contain a "meniscus," a wedge-shaped crescent of solid tissue; one side of the meniscus attaches to the capsule and the free edge extends into the joint. [see Figure 1-8 C]

Box 1-1

---

(3) Structural reinforcement is provided by **ligaments**, tough and inelastic bands of tissue. The anterior and posterior "longitudinal ligaments" travel the length of the spine between vertebral bodies; with the shorter transverse ligaments, they tie adjacent vertebrae together. [see Figure 1-7]

(4) The primary function of **muscles** is not structural support or joining of bone to bone. Unlike ligaments, muscle tissue is elastic and, when stimulated by a nerve, contracts to pull two bony surfaces together. Muscles

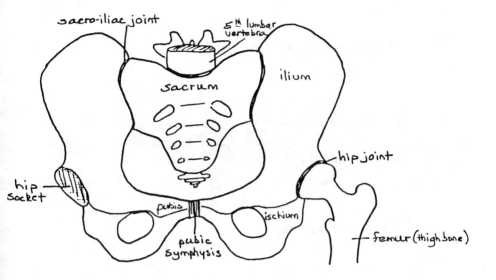

Figure 1-2. The pelvis and sacrum, front view.

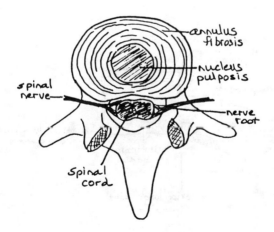

Figure 1-3. Vertebra with disk, spinal cord, nerve roots and spinal nerves, top view.

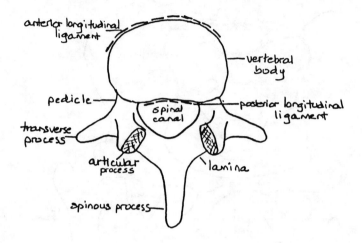

Figure 1-4. Vertebra with longitudinal ligaments, top view.

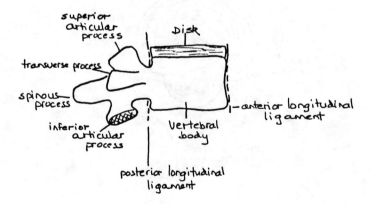

Figure 1-5. Vertebra with disk and longitudinal ligaments, side view.

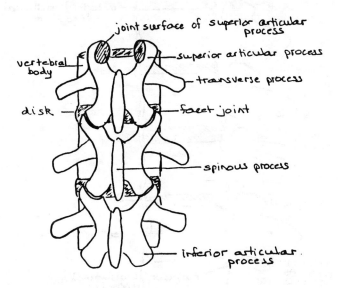

Figure 1-6. Section of the spinal column showing three vertebrae, back view.

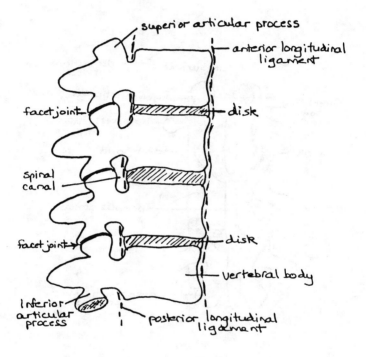

Figure 1-7. Section of the spinal column showing four vertebrae with disks and longitudinal ligaments, side view.

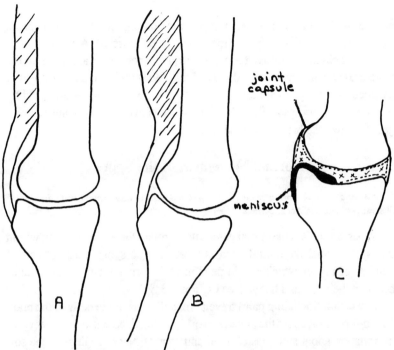

Figure 1-8. (A) Joint in extension with flexor muscle relaxed, side view. (B) Contraction and shortening of flexor muscle to move the joint into flexion. (C) Close-up side view of synovial joint with meniscus; dotted line represents synovial membrane and "x's" represent synovial fluid within the joint space.

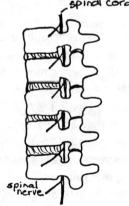

Figure 1-9. Section of the spinal column showing five vertebrae with disks, spinal cord and spinal nerves, side view.

provide strength for movement and postural holding. Some end in tendons, fibrous cords which attach muscle to bone. [see Figure 1-8 A & B]

(5) **Fascia** is connective tissue; it surrounds, permeates and joins all the structures and organs of the body. The brain and spinal cord are also covered by three fascia-type membranes, called "meninges." A liquid produced by the brain, "cerebrospinal fluid," fills the space between the two inner meninges to protect the brain and spinal cord.

Normal Movement of the Spine

"What a piece of work is man! . . . in form and moving how express and admirable!"
Shakespeare, *Hamlet*, Act 2, Scene 2

A passage called the **spinal canal** runs through the spinal column; within this spinal canal the **spinal cord** is located. The spinal cord consists of bundles of nerves which exit in pairs at each vertebra, carrying messages between the brain and body. [see Figures 1-3 & 1-9]

Sensation (including pain) travels from all parts of the body to the brain with information about the physical world. Specialized sensory nerves carry information about sight, taste, smell and sound. Nerve endings in the soft tissues of the body, (the muscles, ligaments, and joint capsules), send the brain information about posture and movement. Feedback from these soft tissues plays a large role in both reflex and voluntary movement. These complex nervous system connections determine the response of the body's musculature to any stimulus, such as a shift in gravity, the decision to move or an injury.

Movement impulses travel in the opposite direction of sensation. Commands initiated in the brain travel down the spinal cord, out the nerve roots and along a nerve to the muscles, causing movement. When stimulated by a nerve impulse, muscles shorten and cause movement at joints by pulling two bony surfaces together. [see Figure 1-8 A & B] "Reflexes" are movements that happen so quickly they initially bypass the brain; a sensation travels inward only as far as the spinal cord, then immediately back to a muscle. For example, when someone touches a hot stove, her hand is jerked away before her brain can register pain.

Normal movement is limited by the shape, depth, type, and angle of joints, their ligamentous and muscular support and the presence of surrounding structures; due to all these factors different joints of the spine have different ranges of motion. The muscles that cross the small joints of the spine can cause movement in three planes.

* flexion/extension (bending and straightening)
* lateral flexion (bending away from the body's midline)
* rotation (twisting)

These facet joint movements are under voluntary control. Another kind of movement is called "joint play"; this refers to the small involuntary movements that occur within a joint in response to outside forces.

Spinal Dysfunction

"What we take for a cure is often just a momentary rally or a new form of the disease."
Duc Francois LaRochefoucauld

Back pain is a symptom present in a wide variety of health problems. Before assuming that a patient is one of the estimated 85-90 percent who fall into the "low back syndrome" category,[1,2] a physician may need to consider and rule out any number of conditions or diseases. These can be differentiated from the low back syndromes, because most can eventually be diagnosed through radiographic, laboratory or other tests. Examples are bone tumors, rheumatoid arthritis and spinal tuberculosis.

When the diagnosable diseases have been ruled out, some patients are left without a firm diagnosis; others are diagnosed with a syndrome involving pathology of one of the following spinal structures.

1) Intervertebral Disks – Commonly called slipped disks, this condition results when the inner part of the disk pushes through the outer fibers. If this causes a bulging, it is called a **prolapsed disk**; if a fragment pushes all the way through, it is a **ruptured disk**. Ruptured disks may or may not cause nerve root compression. [see Figure 1-10]

2) Facet Joints – The moveable joints linking the vertebrae are the facets. They are subject to a variety of **facet joint dysfunction** such as sprain, inflammation, arthritis and instability. One of these joints may also become displaced and jammed; when this happens the soft tissues of the joint can be pinched. This is called acute locked back syndrome. [see Figure 1-11]

3) Soft Tissue – The non-structural parts of the spine include muscles, tendons, ligaments and fascia. Injuries to muscles or ligaments are called **strains** and **sprains**, respectively. When a muscle stays tightened to protect itself or other structures, it is in **spasm**. The role of fascia, or connective

tissue, as a primary site of back pain is gaining popularity, but is still controversial.

4) The Whole Spine – Degenerative disk disease, arthritis and degenerative disease of the spine are all terms used to describe the changes of aging; these affect vertebrae, disks, facet joints and soft tissues. The combination of these degenerative changes is called **spondylosis**. [see Figure 1-12]

5) Sacro-iliac Joints – The SI joint has limited movement, but it can become wedged and irritated, especially if it is excessively mobile to begin with. This syndrome is called **sacro-iliac joint dysfunction**.

6) Piriformis Muscle – This condition also involves soft tissue, but is localized to a specific muscle. If the piriformis muscle goes into spasm, it can compress the sciatic nerve, causing both localized and referred pain. This describes the **piriformis syndrome**. [see Figure 1-13]

There are many who think years of poor posture has the most dramatic impact on causing any of the six syndromes and is the chief culprit in most low back and neck problems. Poor posture is known to predispose disks, muscles and SI joints to injury and to speed the degenerative process of the spine.

The many structures of the spine are interrelated and injury to one can initiate pain and dysfunction in the others. Experts on back pain disagree widely on which is usually the site of the primary pathology. With six specific syndromes to choose from, one would expect that identifying the problem would be routine. Many factors complicate the issue. [see Box 1-2] Due to individual differences and the interrelatedness of spinal structures, pinpointing the site of primary pathology may be impossible. However, specific symptoms are usually associated with specific spinal structures; for many patients careful evaluation can lead to a definitive diagnosis. The more accurate the understanding of the symptoms, the easier it is to select the appropriate treatment approach. With or without a clear diagnosis, the doctor and patient must eventually decide on a plan to relieve and manage the patient's back pain.

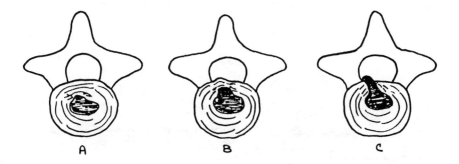

Figure 1-10. Increasingly severe levels of disk dysfunction, top view. (A) Tearing of inner annular fibers. (B) Tearing of inner and outer annular fibers with bulging of annulus into spinal canal. (C) Rupture of annular fibers with extrusion of nuclear material into the spinal canal.

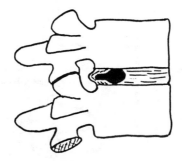

Section of vetebral column showing 2 vertebrae with a prolapsed disk bulging into the spinal canal and compressing the posterior longitudinal ligament, side view.

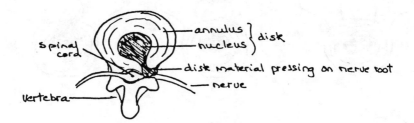

Vertebra, top view, with a ruptured disk compressing a nerve root.

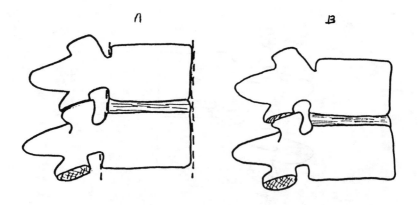

Figure 1-11. (A) Section of the spinal column showing 2 vertebrae, side view. (B) Subluxation (displacement) of the facet joint causing narrowing of the spinal canal, with possible pinching of the soft tissues of the joint or entrapment of a spinal nerve against the vertebral body or disk.

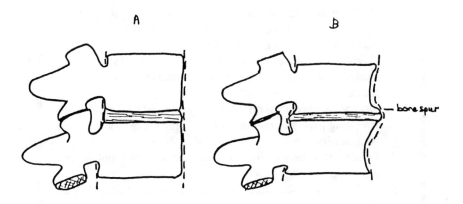

Figure 1-12. (A) Section of the spinal column showing 2 vertebrae, side view. (B) Spondylosis of spinal column, (flattened and misshapen vertebral bodies, flattened disks, worn down and jammed facet joints, narrowed spinal canal, stretched ligaments and development of bone spurs).

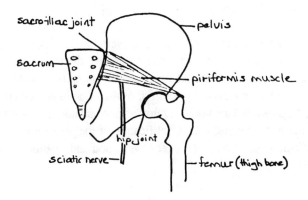

Figure 1-13. Pelvis, sacrum and thigh bone, back view, with piriformis muscle and sciatic nerve.

27

> 1) Different distinct syndromes can yield the same symptoms.
> 2) Syndromes producing characteristic symptoms may occasionally present in an atypical way.
> 3) When facet joints are involved, the disk is affected and vice versa.
> 4) Muscle spasm may accompany spinal pain no matter what the cause.
> 5) Degenerative changes on x-rays may be unrelated to pain.
> 6) Radiating pain does not necessarily imply nerve root compression.
> 7) Pathology in one structure can cause mechanical problems in any weight-bearing joint.
> 8) Piriformis muscle spasm can cause sacro-iliac strain and vice versa.
> 9) Irritated tissue in a sclerotome (deep tissues innervated by the same spinal nerve) can cause irritation in all tissues of that sclerotome.
> 10) Sclerotomes and dermatomes (skin area innervated by the same spinal nerve) do not correspond exactly.
> **Box 1-2**

Key Points - The Normal Back

The back is a complex unit made up of vertebrae, disks, facet joints, sacro-iliac joints, ligaments, muscles and connective tissue. Each structure assists in one or both of the dual functions of the spine – stability and movement. Back pain can be the result of dysfunction in any one of these structures; diagnosis and treatment requires an understanding of their normal functions and interrelationships. Identification of the primary site of pain can be difficult, even impossible; every evaluation and treatment must be individualized.

Footnotes

1 *The Back Letter*, Vol. 4, No. 3
2 Richard DonTigny, "Function and Pathomechanics of the Sacroiliac Joint"

Chapter 2 - Acute Versus Chronic Pain

"Illness is the most heeded of doctors: to goodness and wisdom we only make promises; pain we obey." Marcel Proust

Acute pain is a normal, protective response to alert the body to possible tissue damage. It is an unpleasant sensation, from discomfort to agony, caused by the stimulation of specialized nerve endings. Pain is primarily associated with physical injury, but since pain is a perception it may not be proportional or even directly related to an injury. The experience of hurting is a composite of physical, intellectual, emotional, motivational and situational reactions. Factors other than tissue damage may directly affect the severity, tolerance and persistence of symptoms. In addition, pain does not necessarily correspond to the damaged area; it may move or change, and may or may not follow expected patterns of radiation. These are among the many reasons that pain may not be an accurate measure of the location and severity of an injury. They all need to be taken into consideration in the diagnosis and treatment of back pain.

Pain: An Unreliable Indicator of Pathology

"Pain is perception. Therefore all pain is in the brain." American Osteopathic Association [2]

1) Pain is highly subjective and influenced by emotional, intellectual and situational factors. A child may perceive the pain of a skinned knee differently in the presence of friends than in the company of his doting grandparents.

2) Accuracy of pain localization depends on nearness of the injury to the body surface. The pain from a rapped shin bone is well defined compared to the diffuse ache of an intestinal upset.

3) Pain perception does not necessarily correspond to the site of stimulation; pain can be referred to other structures. During a heart attack, severe pain may be felt down the left arm.

4) Different structures have different sensitivities to pain. [see Box 2-1]

Pain Sensitivity in Spinal Tissues

Some spinal structures are essentially without pain receptors; these include intervertebral disks, cartilage, vertebral bodies (unless invaded by cancer) and nerve roots. Pain responsive tissue (in the approximate order of sensitivity) includes the periosteum (outer covering of bone), joint capsules, synovial lining, ligaments, subchondral bone (bone which lies beneath cartilage), tendons, nerves and nerve sheaths, fascia (connective tissue), cortical bone (bone which composes the outer layer of the shaft) and muscles.

In back dysfunction, the structures that usually give rise to pain are the anterior and posterior longitudinal ligaments, the outer covering of the nerve roots (the dura), the spinal muscles, the fascia of the muscles, the facet joints and the sacro-iliac joints.

Box 2-1

---

5) Severe pain in one structure can block pain from another structure. When someone stubs a toe, the pain from a headache is temporarily forgotten.

6) Pain is blocked by sensory stimulation. When an individual bangs her head, her tendency is to rub it. [see Box 2-2]

Gate Control Theory

Pain travels in small nerve fibers; it is usually blocked at the spinal cord by a steady volume of large fiber (sensory) impulses. When a strong enough painful stimulus occurs, the message of pain from the small pain fibers blocks the large fiber transmission to reach the brain and consciousness. Pain which would normally reach someone's awareness can in turn be blocked by increased levels of sensory stimulation. This view of pain perception is called gate control theory and is discussed in Chapter 5 under "Acupuncture and TENS."

Box 2-2

---

7) Pain can radiate, following nerve, muscle or embryological patterns of distribution.[8] "Sciatica" is felt as pain down the back of the leg, but it usually indicates a problem in the lumbo-sacral spine.

8) Painful structures can increase pain perception or can block pain in other structures from the same embryological segment. [see Box 2-3]

Embryological Pain Patterns

Pain patterns associated with deep injury may be related to the embryological development of the musculoskeletal system. When one structure is injured, other structures which originated in the fetus from the same mass of tissue are affected. The results may include an embryological pattern of increased muscle tone, hyperactive reflexes and increased skin sensitivity.[8]

Box 2-3

---

9) Pain perception can depend on the temporal or spatial summation of stimuli. An individual can comfortably perform may repetitions of a specific exercise and then suddenly feel pain the next time the motion is repeated.

10) Pain is inconsistent and may change in location and severity. The ache of an arthritic hip may wax and wane throughout the day for no apparent reason.

11) Pain is strongly influenced by the "placebo effect," the relief of symptoms caused only by the belief that one is receiving a pain-relieving treatment. The

placebo effect may work through the production of "endorphins," the body's natural pain killers. (Endorphins are discussed in Chapter 5.)

12) Pain can persist after its organic cause has been treated and thought to be corrected. A whiplash injury may result in chronic pain despite the fact that no evidence of tissue damage remains.

The Classification of Pain

"The Greeks viewed pain as an experience resulting from some failure in the right process of living." Steven Brena, MD [4]

There are three kinds of pain. Back pain can fit into any one of these categories; it is one type of pain that does not necessarily correspond to the site of tissue damage or extent of an injury.

1) **Transient pain** is of short duration and serves as a warning signal, such as with a stubbed toe or from touching a hot stove.

2) **Acute pain** is secondary to specific tissue damage such as with a sprained ankle or stomach ulcer.

3) **Chronic pain** is caused by persistent disease such as rheumatoid arthritis, or it is a condition which lasts beyond the expected recovery time.

The type of pain which causes the most puzzlement and frustration to both patient and practitioner is chronic pain, where the pain persists after the physical cause has been treated and considered corrected. A back condition becomes "chronic" after a maximum of six months; some call it chronic after three months or even six weeks. The pain is constant, waxing and waning but seldom disappearing, and doesn't respond to treatment. To all appearances the patient's clinical picture improves with no remaining evidence of injury, but the symptoms do not. As much as 35 percent of the adult population may experience chronic pain for a significant period of their lives; 10-15 percent of Americans may suffer from pain at any one time.[3] Back pain is the most common kind of chronic pain.[9]

The Causes of Chronic Pain

"We have no business calling a patient a malingerer just because we cannot find a physical basis for his pain or because he's had it for a very long period." Stanley Paris, PT[8]

It is not known why some people's pain lasts far beyond the expected recovery period. Five possible explanations follow.

1) Chronic pain may be explained as continuing pathology of spinal structures which has not yet been identified. Given the difficulty in diagnosing back pain, this is not an unreasonable option.

2) Chronic pain may result from a change in the nervous system's transmission of pain messages; cells that normally fire once start to respond excessively to minor, innocuous stimuli.[5] The continuing barrage of pain impulses eventually may break down the brain or spinal cord mechanisms which would normally block perception of minor pain impulses.[4] The pain becomes less and less associated with a physical basis as time goes by.[11]

3) The body's physical response to acute injury can perpetuate chronic pain. Back muscles go into spasm to splint and protect a spinal injury, causing a build-up of toxins, decreased blood flow and eventually stiffness and reduced activity; all of these conditions can themselves produce pain. Emotional responses to being in pain also increase muscular tension. The persistence of symptoms is exhausting, but sleep is disturbed by the pain and anxiety, increasing fatigue. All these factors create a cycle of anxiety, muscle tension and pain, each perpetuating the others.[1,4,5,6,10]

4) Chronic pain may be due to the postural adjustments which are made in response to an acute injury; these myofascial compensations are made in an attempt to relieve pain and may then become habit. Postural muscles no longer relax or contract efficiently and are not recruited in their normal patterns of movement. The original injury may be resolved, but the pain is perpetuated by the postural dysfunction.[7]

5) Many practitioners specializing in the treatment of chronic pain believe that its explanation lies in a patient's emotional make-up. The theory that chronic pain is psychogenic versus somatogenic, (originating in the mind versus the body), or that it is perpetuated by emotional factors is well-established in the chronic pain field.

A generalized explanation of chronic pain applied to back dysfunction might be as follows. Chronic back pain usually begins with injury or strain of spinal structures, but it becomes a disorder in and of itself with both physical and psychological characteristics. Normal responses to physical pain, (muscle spasm, restricted activity, postural compensations, anxiety, depression and fatigue), can initiate a cycle which helps to perpetuate the pain. Eventually, pain perception may be maintained by the nervous system with little input form the original site of injury. Whatever is happening on a physical level, the pain has stopped serving a useful purpose in protecting the body.[6,10]

Key Points - Acute Versus Chronic Pain

Pain is a normal protective mechanism of the body which signals potential tissue damage. However, pain is not a reliable guide to the location and extent of an injury. Chronic pain occurs when symptoms persist long after an injury, with no remaining physical evidence of tissue damage. Different theories are put forth explaining the development of chronic pain.

Footnotes

1   Edward Abraham, *Freedom from Back Pain: An Orthopedist's Self-Help Guide*
2   American Osteopathic Association, informational literature
3   "Approaches to Musculoskeletal Problems: Focus on the Low Back" Symposium, Jane Derebery
4   Steven Brena, *Chronic Pain: America's Hidden Epidemic*
5   Rene Cailliet, *Low Back Pain Syndrome*
6   Barbara Headley, *Chronic Pain: Life Out of Balance*
7   Barbara Headley, "Postural Homeostasis"
8   Stanley Paris, *The Spine*
9   Jo Solet, "Low Back Pain – An Overview"
10   Richard Sternbach, *Pain Patients: Traits and Treatments*
11   David Zinman, "Focus on Back Pain"

Chapter 3 -
The Professional View

Effects of Pain on Personality

"Chronic symptoms in compensable cases should be considered psychogenic [originating in the mind] *unless the failure to recover can be clearly shown to be a normal response to injury."* Jane Derebery, MD and William Tullis, MD[7]
"Treat the patient as if he has a real problem until proven otherwise." Duane Saunders, PT[11]

As pain continues, a patient becomes more desperate and may risk therapies with possible side-effects, drug addiction, unnecessary surgeries and potentially harmful quackery. A variety of diagnoses and unsuccessful treatments reinforces the belief that the condition is serious and untreatable. Such a situation strains the doctor-patient relationship. Trying to contribute to the diagnostic effort, the patient reports small, probably insignificant symptoms; this may cause the doctor to think the patient is complaining about everything. Not knowing what to do makes it hard for patients to take control and this may be seen as dependent behavior. Patients are often asked about "secondary gains" which seems to imply a suspicion of malingering. Even for those who normally get plenty of support and enjoy their work, secondary benefits, such as sympathy, attention and decreased responsibility, do exist.

Under these circumstances, people are apt to demonstrate any of the following responses:

- muscle tension
- anxiety
- depression
- inability to take control
- stress
- restricted activity
- poor sleeping
- seeking help from a variety of sources
- use of medications
- trials of unproven or risky treatments
- belief that the condition is more serious than it is
- reporting of numerous symptoms or complaints
- presence of secondary gains

These reactions are normal for people suffering unresolved pain and dysfunction; however, without physical evidence of injury, they may be viewed by health practitioners as indications that the pain is psychogenic.

Every patient with back pain of physical origin eventually undergoes a secondary change in personality; the chronic pain experience has a marked and deep effect. One study concludes that if pain persists for more than three months, the psychological make-up of the patient changes and complete recovery is impaired;[6] another that workers sick-listed for more than three months have virtually no chance of recovering normal function.[3] When symptoms go on for months, the patient develops emotional overlay typical of psychogenic pain patients; chronic pain is even said by some to cause emotional disturbance.[13] It can only be speculated that chronic pain patients formerly had more normal-looking psychological profiles, but life histories support the fact that most functioned well before the onset of their pain.[13]

There is often a great fear on the part of patients that chronic back problems will be judged to be emotionally based. Although emotional and physical factors cannot be isolated, both patients and practitioners worry about chronic pain being psychogenic. The conclusions drawn influence how patients feel about themselves and how practitioners treat their patients.

Effects of Personality on Pain

"Successful treatment depends on recognizing that the primary problem is emotional." [7]

Many experts in the field of back pain believe that personality traits have a major role in determining which patients will develop chronic symptoms.

- *"The vast majority of patients will have a psychological explanation for their continued physical misery."* [7]

- *"Explore why you don't want to get better."* [1]

- *"The doctor has a responsibility to detect and treat pathology; the patient has a responsibility to provide organic pathology to justify treatment."* [13]

- *"Pain is a socially acceptable excuse for self-doubt and the inability to cope with life."* [5]

- *"Only a small proportion of patients with chronic pain are too engaged in their lives to constantly seek answers, proud of their independence and ability to deal with their handicap."* [13]

- *"The vast majority are persons with pre-existing psychosocial impairments."* [9]

- *"50-70 percent of chronic symptoms are psychological in origin."* [2]

- *"In sum, the patient tyrannizes those at home by avoiding his responsibilities, controlling their behavior and getting payoffs, while he lies around feeling sorry for himself."* [13]

- One author's standard for pain tolerance is exemplified in a story in which a man having his gangrenous leg amputated without anesthesia thanks the surgeon effusively. The author's comment—*"What an impressive example of self-control and positive thinking!"* [5]

Pain which persists long after an injury and which is reinforced by the environment is thought to be associated with a clear psychological profile and specific behaviors; the name for this combination of circumstances is **chronic pain syndrome.** Some patients are thought to be at risk for the development of chronic pain syndrome. Those who are low in self-esteem, mildly depressed, anxious, angry, dependent or susceptible to hysteria are more apt to believe in the seriousness and hopelessness of the condition and perpetuate the chronic pain cycle. Such people have poor coping skills and are often unable to problem solve in order to meet their needs in healthy ways. They may respond to stress with physical symptoms instead of dealing with their problems. If they were success-fully treated for their symptoms, they would have to learn new behaviors, so they're highly committed to their physical complaints and resist giving them up. The person with chronic pain syndrome is especially likely to resist change. [see Box 3-1]

Psychological Testing

Tools such as the "Minnesota Multiphasic Personality Inven-tory" have been used to try to determine if pain is psychogenic. As with other pain assessment tests, there is controversy concerning reliability of results. On testing, chronic pain has been associated with "neuroticism," a greater than normal concern with physical symptoms.[13] Low scores in "perceived control" are present in those with high levels of pain and dysfunction; however, "active coping" scores do not correlate with better pain adjustment.[3] Some re-searchers rely heavily on pain drawings to identify psychogenic pain patients; the amount of body surface affected and location of the pain are sketched in on a body chart by the patient. It is far from unanimous that a pain drawing is a strong indicator of psychological illness; the connection has been said to be inconsistent and unreli-able.[4]

Box 3-1

Personality Traits and History Associated
with the Risk of Developing Chronic Pain

- poor self-image
- hostility or anger
- pessimistic outlook on life
- inability to fantasize
- low threshold for pain
- poor social relationships
- sex problems
- self-preoccupation
- GI symptoms
- dysfunctional family
- insomnia
- recent family or personal crisis
- workaholic tendencies
- substance abuse
- neurotic, moody, irritable or anxious personality
- overreaction to minor incidents
- frustration or discouragement
- poor coping skills, adaptability and problem-solving
- indecisiveness or lack of assertiveness
- low activity level, poor physical conditioning and fatigue
- mental dullness and unresponsiveness
- dependence on others for emotional and financial support
- rationalization of failures and mistakes
- history of other chronic problems
- family history of depression
- cultural factors such as tendency to be emotional
- family reinforcement of dependency
- job dissatisfaction, absenteeism

Symptoms or History Indicating Pain is Psychogenic

- use of pain as an excuse
- withdrawal from social life
- acceptance of powerlessness
- guilt
- increasingly low activity level

- injury which is compensable
- constant obsession with pain
- doctor shopping
- multiple surgeries
- self-pity
- despair
- denial of emotional problems
- expectation of failure in treatment
- unresolved anger at someone or something that caused the pain
- use of pain to manipulate and control
- withdrawal from sex
- increased number of hysterical outbursts
- change in interpersonal relationships
- depression and disinterest in usual activities
- pending litigation (often with support of attorney)
- use of exaggerations to describe pain ("excruciating")
- verbalization of extensive and varied physical complaints
- seeking justification and reaffirmation of problems
- symptoms with no possible correlations to physical cause
- grimacing or exaggerated gestures
- misuse, overuse or reliance on medications
- family conflict in which a relative is accused of not helping
- unwillingness to consider alternate employment

The motivating factors for psychogenic pain patients are thought to be financial compensation, attention, avoidance of stressful situations and responsibility, avoidance of work, excuse for failure, addiction, confounding doctors or the sick role itself. Although this seems to imply an intentional rouse on the part of the patient, actual malingering (pretending to have pain) is uncommon.[10,12] Usually chronic pain syndrome is an unconscious process and the pain is very real. When pain is relieved by counseling or stress reduction treatment, this in no way invalidates the pain experience.

Workers' Compensation Patients

"The patient loses his amateur (acute patient) standing when he accepts financial reward for his patienthood." Richard Sternbach, MD [13]

Opinions concerning the effects of personality on chronic pain seem doubly strong for the patient injured on the job. Low back pain accounts for 35 percent of compensable disabling injuries.[7] Financial gain, (or even revenge), is seen as the motivating factor for the continuation of disability. The workers' compensation system financially rewards the patient for pain, especially with back symptoms where disability is hard to prove or disprove. The legal system also contributes to delayed recovery through the lengthy claims process. Research supports the importance of compensation relative to chronic pain. Patients receiving compensation have a disproportionate amount of disability and delay in recovery, showing 33 percent less objective evidence and 44 percent less long-term improvement than those not getting compensation.[7] Doctors are recommended to assume that a physical explanation is the least likely cause of delayed recovery in compensable patients.[7]

Whether or not financial compensation is involved, the contribution of emotional factors to the continuation of symptoms must be judged objectively for each individual patient. Any of the following may be true.
• Pain is causing secondary emotional stress.
• Stress is prolonging or producing pain.
• Pain is present with no psychological disorder.
• Pain is present with a concurrent psychiatric diagnosis.

A practitioner does a patient a great disservice by automatically assuming that a lack of objective findings proves that tension or neurosis is responsible for the pain; this reaction can only contribute to the patient's emotional stress. On the other hand, patients should be willing to examine the role of stress without defensiveness or guilt. Tension reducing treatment is a valid approach for many people with back pain. Referral to a psychiatrist or counselor does not mean the pain is imagined or that the patient is mentally ill. Such a referral is appropriate when anxiety or depression interfere with treatment, when interpersonal relationships are threatened, during a personal crisis or when social isolation or drug abuse result.

41

Chapter 3

Key Points - The Professional View

Many experts believe that patients with a specific psychological profile are especially at risk for the development of chronic pain. Symptoms are thought to be psychologically induced as a maladaptive reaction to stress. However, "despite strong opinions to the contrary, no definitive chronic pain personality can be identified."[8]

Whatever originally causes and perpetuates back pain, it is complicated by emotional overlay; chronic pain has a marked and deep effect on every patient. Seeking help for the stress caused by chronic pain is a treatment option that patients should consider without defensiveness. On the other hand, health care providers should not automatically assume that chronic back pain is psychological in origin. Treatment should meet both the physical and emotional needs of the patient and to do so must be individualized.

Footnotes

1   Edward Abraham, *Freedom from Back Pain: An Orthopedist's Self-Help Guide*
2   "Approaches to Musculoskeletal Problems: Focus on the Low Back" Symposium, Jane Derebery
3   *The Back Letter*, Vol. 4, No. 3
4   *The Back Letter*, Vol. 4, No. 4
5   Steven Brena, *Chronic Pain: America's Hidden Epidemic*
6   Rene Cailliet, *Low Back Pain Syndrome*
7   Derebery & Tullis, "Delayed Recovery in the Patient with a Work Compensable Injury"
8   Barbara Headley, "Pain Vs. Suffering"
9   Tom Mayer, "Rehabilitation of the Patient with Spinal Pain"
10 John Rice, et al., "Low Back Pain: The Rheumatologist's View"
11 Duane Saunders, *Evaluation, Treatment and Prevention of Musculoskeletal Disorders*
12 Carl Sherman, "The Medicolegal Thicket of Low Back Disability"
13 Richard Sternbach, *Pain Patients: Traits and Treatments*

Chapter 4 -
The Patient's View

"Those who do not feel pain seldom think that it is felt." Dr. Samuel Johnson

Chronic pain invades and threatens every part of an individual's life. The period spent searching for a diagnosis and cure is a state of limbo; life is on hold, centered around the hope for relief. Between three to six months following the onset of pain, a person's status suddenly changes. The pain is still present and the individual is still waiting for life to return to normal, but to the medical world that person is now a "chronic pain patient".

As discussed in Chapter 3, it is a widely held belief that the majority of people with chronic pain have "pre-existing psychosocial impairments."[2] Therefore, when six months have elapsed with no improvement, patients may start being treated differently by their practitioners. The sympathetic, caring attitude of friends and family can also gradually dissolve over time; others may come to doubt the pain is real. Patients feel trapped in a no-win situation.

If they keep looking for a cure and refuse to succumb to the pain, they are in denial and can't accept reality; if they stop looking for a cure and make adjustments, they are quitters and are accepting the sick role. Meanwhile they receive advice from family, friends, acquaintances, strangers, books, articles and TV talk shows. It is meant to be helpful or inspiring, but can be perceived as confusing, judgmental or demoralizing.

"Expert" opinions to the contrary, there are many active, enthusiastic people whose chronic pain interrupted challenging, rewarding work. Their lives and futures have been turned upside down; they often don't know what's wrong or why or if they'll ever regain their previous levels of health. Careers, relationships and self-images are rocked. Whatever secondary gains may be inherent in this situation, they don't begin to make up for the losses.

Any kind of pain is difficult to tolerate in the following circumstances:
- when the pain is overwhelming
- when the pain continues indefinitely with no end in sight
- when the source of the pain is unknown
- when a person feels unable to control the pain
- when serious illness hasn't been ruled out as the cause of the pain
- when the pain is meaningless, unrelated to any action or seemingly due to chance
- when physicians do not validate the pain, causing patients to distrust their perceptions of reality.

All of these factors may exist with chronic back pain. The constancy and endlessness of the symptoms are exhausting and interfere with coping skills. The result is a situation which causes feelings of helplessness and hopelessness.

Three major parts of a chronic pain person's life are deeply affected – activities, relationships with other people and feelings about oneself. What follows is an examination of the impact chronic pain has on these three areas. Each section concludes with the comments of individuals who live with disabling back conditions and who answered this survey question, "What has been the most difficult aspect for you of having chronic pain?"

Feelings About Self

"You may start to cry at the most unexpected time and for the smallest reasons." Sefra
Pitzele[3]

Chronic pain threatens a person's self-image, self-esteem and self-confidence. People are diminished by a loss of function; their self-images are
often defined by abilities and roles. Since back problems severely curtail
the normal range of activities, people can no longer fulfill their roles; they
are incomplete, no longer themselves. The feeling of uselessness radical-
ly diminishes the sense of being a valuable, contributing member of
family, society and life. One's perception of the future, upon which hope
is based, is suddenly unclear.[1]

What has been the most difficult aspect for you of having chronic pain?

- *"Recognizing that I will never be like I used to be."* Eleanor C.,
  Meadowbrook, Pennsylvania

- *"Not knowing when it will start or stop; it seems to be out of my
  control."* Adie C., Mendham, New Jersey

- *"Treatment failures."* Deborah M., Trenton, New Jersey

- *"Adjusting to an invisible disability, accepting dependency and life-
  long limitations."* Audrey S., Old Orchard Beach, Maine

- *"Having prolonged periods of self-pity."* Evelyn F., Bath, Maine

- *"Everything takes longer to do and is an effort."* Roberta E., Cincin-
  nati, Ohio

- *"Being irritable and impatient and the loss of control."* Audrey A.,
  Brunswick, Maine

- *"Feelings of uselessness, the inability to concentrate, immobility."*
  Audrey S., Old Orchard Beach, Maine

- *"Needing to adapt; not being able to do lots of things I once could do
  and still want to do."* Audrey A., Brunswick, Maine

- *"The difficulty in planning ahead."* Robert N., Abbington, Pennsylvania

- *"Not knowing the future."* Deborah M., Trenton, New Jersey

- *"The inability to sleep well."* Eleanor C., Meadowbrook, Pennsylvania
- *"Feeling like a wimp."* Audrey A., Brunswick, Maine
- *"I feel like I aged suddenly and dramatically."* Sandra G., Yarmouth, Maine
- *"Depression is probably the most difficult battle to surmount."* Audrey S., Old Orchard Beach, Maine
- *"I'm tired of hurting every day."* Susan B., Brunswick, Maine

Activities

"I discovered myself wanting to play tennis and go on a long bike ride soon after I began feeling my acute sense of loss. Never mind that I rarely played tennis before and avoided bike riding by letting the air out of my tires!" Sefra Pitzele[3]

Options and choices are limited when back pain becomes chronic. Traditional ways of working and having fun are suddenly out of reach. Not only are leisure-time activities restricted, but there may suddenly be too much leisure.

1) **Shopping** can be a major hurdle; it entails standing in line, finding a place to park to minimize walking, stooping and bending to reach items or unload a grocery cart, trying on clothes, even struggling with a heavy door to get into a store.

2) **Driving** is considered one of the worst activities for the back, but most Americans depend on their cars for mobility. Adapting cars to minimize stress on the back can be expensive, especially if a new car is the only way to get a contoured or adjustable seat, a hand brake, sufficient leg room, power steering or an automatic transmission. Public transportation involves standing, walking, waiting, carrying bundles and often sitting in uncomfortable seats.

3) **Entertainment** often means sitting in restaurants, theaters or at sporting events. Restaurant chairs may be uncomfortable and slow service means a prolonged period of sitting. This is also true when watching a movie, play or concert. Sporting events, already off limits for participation, usually require prolonged standing or attempting to cope with bleachers.

Any activity now requires planning ahead; unexpected delays or last-minute errands can threaten a carefully planned schedule. The need to balance physical activity with rest and to get priority tasks completed takes the spontaneity out of one's daily life. With physical resources limited, it is difficult to add a spur-of-the-moment activity without canceling another. Some activities are abandoned altogether; the ones that used to be done with family and friends are especially missed. And while it is necessary to preplan for the week ahead, it is impossible to plan for the more distant future. The person with chronic pain doesn't know how he will feel next week or how disabled she might be next year.

What Has Been the Most Difficult Aspect for you of Having Chronic Pain?

- *"Not being able to do physical activities without paying for it later."* Pauline M., Tenants Harbor, Maine
- *"Worrying about sitting – in meetings, traveling."* Eve. F., Watertown, Massachusetts
- *"The loss of spontaneity in activities."* Barbara Y., Brunswick, Maine
- *"Having to hire people to do work for me that I'd rather be doing myself, and could do better before."* Eleanor C., Meadowbrook, Pennsylvania
- *"Making rest time."* Barbara Y., Brunswick, Maine
- *"Giving up the physical activities I like."* Eve F., Watertown, Massachusetts

Relationships

"Close to 75 percent of all marriages in which one partner has a chronic medical condition fail." Sefra Pitzele[3]

Back pain not only changes one's self-image and activity level, it can also have a dramatic impact on relations with others. That part of oneself that exists in the context of the social and political realms may be lost. Society places a premium on the needs and wishes of bright, healthy types; this influences the way people with disabilities are viewed and how they view themselves. Chronic back pain can push individuals into isolation either through their own perceptions or through the reactions of other people. The following scenarios are not uncommon.

1) A person with chronic pain keeps her feelings surrounding the pain to herself out of fear of boring others or because others really do lose interest.

2) Feelings of diminished self-worth damage his self-confidence in social situations.

3) Feeling guilty about the excessive demands placed on friends and family, she refuses their help in order to salvage some independence, thereby becoming more isolated.

4) Too much help and sympathy from friends cause his relationships to center around his health problem; his friendships no longer seem based on mutual give and take.

5) Due to immobility, medications and depression, her physical appearance may change; even if it doesn't, she feels less worthy overall and this makes her feel less attractive and less confident.

6) Feeling that there is nothing to talk about but complaints, he avoids calling his friends and asking for support; sometimes there is just not enough energy left for reaching out.

7) Back pain is often a "hidden handicap"; she looks normal so others don't understand why she's asking for help, moving so slowly, resting so much or over-reacting to little things. Other people have no concept of the effort required to do something as simple as grocery shopping.

8) "How are you?" is the most common greeting in our society; it usually means 'hello,' but flusters him. "Do they really want to know how I am? I should say I'm fine, but I don't feel fine."

9) Large social events are difficult; it is impossible to mingle and find a comfortable position at the same time. She can use adaptive equipment, but this focuses attention on her disability and may make the other guests uncomfortable. Ignoring her physical limits increases the pain level to the point that she can't enjoy the party. She decides to avoid large gatherings altogether.

10) Some people are uncomfortable around someone with a disability and don't know how to relate to him. Certain friendships may end, just when he feels most in need of support.

11) There are people who dislike or disapprove of pain; society places a high value on fortitude. Because she has succumbed to a chronic back problem, she is viewed as weak and dependent.

12) Many people minimize back problems, believing that everyone has

them to one extent or another. Their stories about others in worse straits make him feel like a baby and that no one understands how hard he's trying. It hurts to be told, "Stop feeling sorry for yourself!" Comparing himself to others with worse disabilities may put his problem in perspective, but his losses are still significant when compared to how he used to be.

13) She is subjected to an avalanche of well-intentioned advice, much of it pressed on her by people who are sure they have the answers. She is exceptionally vulnerable to this kind of pressure since she hasn't been successful in curing herself. She is aware that she knows more about her own situation than anyone else, but still wonders, "Should I try that?"

14) Some who are uncomfortable with other people's health problems try to convince him (and themselves) that it's not so bad. They insist that he look on the bright side all the time; they are unable to just listen and allow him to express his frustrations. They tend to say things like, "You look great; you must be feeling better!"; this encourages a stiff upper lip and keeps him from sharing his true feelings.

15) One viewpoint expressed is that "everything's for the best" or that the pain "was meant to be." Another particularly galling philosophy is that the pain was "chosen" in a previous life.

What Has Been the Most Difficult Aspect for You of Having Chronic Pain?

- *"Feeling as though no one really knows how I feel and not being able to communicate well about it."* Susan B., Brunswick, Maine

- *"Having an invisible problem when I look healthy; being torn between wanting to convince others I am normal and wanting others to understand my situation and make accommodations gracefully."* Barbara Y., Brunswick, Maine

- *"Feeling like I can't keep up with everyone else."* Susan B., Brunswick, Maine

- *"The loss of spontaneity in my physical relationships."* Deborah M., Trenton, New Jersey

- *"Having the other people around us accept and believe that the pain is real and that we are doing our best to help ourselves."* Jill V., Harpswell, Maine

Chapter 4

- *"Feeling isolated and different than everyone, not normal, and hesitant to socialize."* Susan B., Brunswick, Maine
- *"Stupid comments, unctuous concern and unsolicited health advice."* Barbara Y., Brunswick, Maine
- *"My family still seem to expect me to carry on as usual. I don't know what will happen to me if I get so bad I can't go on as I'm expected to. My family and friends will not let me slow down or quit any of my responsibilities."* Evelyn F., Bath, Maine

Relapse

The leaves turn, the weather changes
All at a distance.
The constancy of pain
Separating me from the outside world,

Draining, sapping, taking my energy
and optimism.
Flares of anger and desolation,
Putting on the capable, cheery face for visitors
which leaves me more exhausted
when they go.

Waiting, waiting . . .
for the doctor to call,
for recovery to begin,
waiting to find out how long this time
before I regain my ration of independence.

Time passes, time wasted,
Seeing the trees, the birds from a distance.
Life permeated by the constant,
hopeless
ache.

Julie Zimmerman

Key Points - The Patient's View

Chronic back pain threatens an individual in the areas of self-image, activities and relationships. The frustrations that accompany this condition are many. In this chapter, people who live with recurrent or chronic disabling back conditions respond to the question, "What has been the most difficult aspect for you of having chronic pain?" Perhaps they can best be summed up by the following comments.

"Backs are a life sentence!" David P., Yarmouth, Maine
"This condition really pisses me off!" Marc Z., Arlington, Virginia

Footnotes

1 Eric Cassel, "The Nature of Suffering and the Goals of Medicine"
2 Tom Mayer, "Rehabilitation of the Patient with Spinal Pain"
3 Sefra Pitzele, *We Are Not Alone: Living with Chronic Illness*

PART 2 - CHRONIC PAIN TREATMENT

Chapter 5 - Pain Inhibition

"There are contrasting and disappointing results from almost every therapy aimed at relieving chronic pain." Steven Brena, MD[1]

Many of the treatments used for both acute and chronic pain patients work by inhibiting the perception of pain. Pain inhibition is a symptomatic, not curative, treatment; it does not remove the factors which originally caused the pain and the effects are relatively short-term.

Endorphins

"Stimulating the body's release of endorphins makes a person feel good and alleviates the stress accumulated during a typical day." Pat Croce[7]

Endorphins are opiate-like derivatives produced by the brain which have a pain-killing effect on the body. They are released in response to tissue damage or trauma. There are treatment approaches which work, at least partially, by stimulating the body to secrete endorphins; they are used for pain inhibition with acute and chronic pain patients.

Endorphins may also be responsible for the "placebo effect," (the relief of symptoms caused only be the belief that one is receiving a pain-relieving treatment). The placebo effect is a major complicating factor in judging the effectiveness of back pain treatments and is higher with back pain than with other kinds of pain. It is not unusual for 30 percent of people with back trouble to feel better after receiving therapy which has no possible pain relieving properties.[6,26]

Exercise

Exercise is considered to be effective in both the prevention of and recovery from back pain.[1] It has multiple benefits and is thought to stimulate the production of endorphins. Studies have found that exercises which do not increase the body's use of oxygen do not effect endorphin response. On the other hand, high intensity exercise results in a dramatic endorphin increase which falls off rapidly when exercise ceases.[12] To optimize physical conditioning, "aerobic" exercises should be selected. Aerobic exercises are so called because they (1) increase the body's use of oxygen and (2) increase heart and lung activity through rhythmic, repetitive activities lasting over 20 minutes. Examples of aerobic activities are running, walking, swimming, dancing and biking. Individuals with chronic back pain, by following a regular fitness program, can prevent or reverse some of the secondary effects of their limitations.[24] A program needs to be tailored so that it is appropriate to each person's specific disability level.

Manual Therapy

Manual therapy is the use of the hands to bring about therapeutic changes within the body; manipulation and mobilization are the two major categories of manual therapy. Manipulation, also called a spinal adjustment, is a sudden thrust of high velocity and small amplitude. Mobilization is a gentler series of rhythmic movements, performed within the patient's available range of motion.[15,18] One way in which manual therapy is thought to relieve pain is through endorphin production, apparently stimulated by the mobilization of the soft tissues and joints of the spine.

Manipulation is controversial and has many critics; some health professionals even feel that its use poses serious health risks.[6,14] What is relevant for chronic pain patients is the research indicating that manipulation has positive short-term effects for some, but that its long-term benefits are questionable.[4,10,16] Manipulation alone seldom cures back pain.

Laughter

Some studies show that humor relieves pain and other symptoms, although the disease itself is still present; laughter can stimulate the production of endorphins.[7] It is also theorized that laughter may reduce the risk of developing health problems, slow their progression or even that it can cure.[22] Another theory is that laughing or assuming a happy facial expression may induce a positive mood, rather than vice versa. What is certain is that humor improves the quality of anyone's life.

Critics of this philosophy are concerned about an exaggeration of the importance of a happy attitude on health. *"Humor tries to make light of death and disability. When the context is the constructive acceptance of reality, that's good. It's not good, however, if humor is used to promote a therapeutic environment in which we are encouraged to abandon rationality, to trust anecdote, to embrace antiscience."*[11]

Acupuncture and TENS

"O, be drest; Stay not for th' other pin!" George Herbert, *The Temple*

The use of vigorous sensory stimulation can produce a sharp decrease in back pain for varying periods of time. Such an effect occurs because the messages from nerves which carry pain impulses are blocked by faster moving impulses from sensory nerves. This is called "gate control theory." [see Box 5-1]

***

Gate Control Theory

Normally, cells in the spinal cord act as censors, moderating the flow of sensory information from the body to the brain. According to gate control theory, impulses from sensory nerves travel faster than pain impulses and "close the gate" so that the slower pain messages do not get to the brain. When a sudden unpleasant stimulus crosses the pain threshold, the gate opens, allowing the sensation to spill over into consciousness.[17,21] Any stimulation that activates sensory nerves, such as rubbing the skin, affects pain perception. When someone bangs his head or raps his shin, he commonly rubs where it hurts; the injury itself is not reduced, but it feels better because rubbing the skin inhibits the pain.

The opposite effect occurs when reduced sensory input increases pain perception. People are normally more aware of any kind of pain at rest; this is because at rest there is decreased visual, joint, muscle and skin stimulation.[21] To use gate control theory to help chronic pain patients, the goal is for maximum stimulation of sensory nerves with minimum pain stimulation.[17] Since people with chronic back problems spend more time resting, one method for inhibiting pain is to gradually increase their activity levels.

Box 5-1

***

The two most common techniques used by professionals for pain inhibition are acupuncture and "transcutaneous electrical nerve stimulation," called TENS. A patient using a TENS unit glues or sticks electrodes on certain skin sites; a mild electrical current, either steady or pulsed, stimulates the skin in order to inhibit pain in the back.[26] The electrical stimulation blocks the transmission of pain impulses. The maximum current which is not unpleasant should be used.[3] TENS units are given to patients to use on their own.

With acupuncture, small needles are inserted into the surface of the skin at selected points; these acupuncture points have a smaller amount of electrical resistance than that of surrounding skin. The needles remain in place for about 20 minutes. Small clips which conduct heat or electricity from a machine are sometimes attached to the ends of the needles; this provides additional kinds of sensory stimulation. The treatment must be performed by a certified acupuncturist, but patients can be taught to perform "acupressure" on themselves; this involves sustained pressure on acupuncture points without the use of needles.

In addition to pain inhibition effects, acupuncture and TENS may also stimulate the body to produce endorphins, its own pain-killers. With the use of these two techniques, some patients report needing shorter periods of stimulation and getting longer periods of relief. This suggests that pain inhibition may have increasingly long-lasting effects.[23]

TENS and acupuncture can help some patients manage pain, but it is not universally successful. A study reported in *The New England Journal of Medicine* states, "We conclude that for patients with chronic low back pain, treatment with TENS is no more effective than treatment with a placebo."[9]

Medications

"The desire to take medicine is perhaps the greatest feature which distinguishes man from animals." Sir William Osler

The medications which are used for people with back pain may be prescribed to inhibit pain, decrease inflammation, relax muscles, decrease tension or elevate mood. They include the following:

NSAIDs (non-steroidal anti-inflammatory drugs) – decrease pain and inflammation [see Box 5-2]

aspirin (salicylates) – decrease pain and inflammation

opiates – decrease pain

barbituates – decrease pain

tranquilizers – decrease emotional tension

anti-depressants – elevate mood [see Box 5-2]

muscle relaxants – decrease muscle tension [see Box 5-2]

NSAIDs, Valium and Anti-Depressants

NSAIDs are routinely prescribed for soft-tissue injuries for weeks or even months; they are thought to contribute to a quicker and better recovery, but research does not uniformly support such an assumption.[2] After an acute injury, inflammation may be excessive and NSAIDs can help to reduce it. However, inflammation is a normal response of the body and probably shouldn't be obliterated.[2] With ongoing back pain the rationale for using NSAIDs is questionable because the cause of the pain may not involve inflammation.

Valium is often prescribed for pain, due to its properties as a muscle relaxant and tranquilizer. However, the drug seems to increase the subjective pain experience and increase feelings of confusion and helplessness.[3] It is now known to have addictive potential with heavy long-term use.

There has recently been success in the use of **anti-depressants** for chronic pain. In one study, patients taking the anti-depressant "amitripyline" became more active with less pain; a comparison group received psychotherapy and, although more productive, reported more pain.[2]

Box 5-2

Certain medications can be helpful during acute episodes and others appropriate for people with chronic pain. However, back pain patients are advised to minimize drug use to avoid the dangers of side effects and physical or emotional addiction. Drug abuse is one of the most devastating complications of chronic pain. Patients can become addicted to pain-killing or other medications; they may even use the pain to justify continued drug use instead of taking more positive measures.[3]

Holistic health practitioners have even stronger objections to the use of medications than the fear of addiction. They believe that synthesized chemicals cannot possibly promote healing or sustain health. Chemical treatments, including antibiotics and immunizations, are thought to meddle with the immune system and interfere with self-healing, causing rather than curing serious health problems.[5]

Surgery and Injections

"Surgery fails completely in 20 percent of patients with low back pain and 60 percent continue to have symptoms." David Imrie, MD[13]

People often believe that surgery is performed when other treatments fail – that it is the drastic but sure answer which will relieve their symptoms. In fact, surgery does not help most back pain patients. It is estimated that only 1 percent of patients with low back pain have true disk ruptures with nerve root compression, which is one of the few indications for an operation.[4] Surgery can be a dramatically successful approach to back pain, but the key is limiting it to appropriate patients with specific pathology. Patients who shop around until they find a surgeon willing to operate have a very good chance of increasing their disability and their pain.

Surgery or injection is occasionally used for patients with severe chronic pain which has not responded to other treatments. The procedure in these cases is not to relieve nerve root compression or correct pathology, but to block pain. [see Box 5-3]

Invasive Procedures for Chronic Pain

1) "Neuroaugmentive" surgery is done for patients with symptoms of chronic dull, aching pain. A device is implanted under the skin; it provides electronic stimulation which blocks the transmission of pain messages.

2) "Deafferation," (such as rhizotomy, cordotomy, dorsal root entry zone radiofrequency lesions or intracranial procedures), controls pain by severing or destroying a sensory nerve. In facet rhizotomy or radiofrequency facet denervation, the sensory nerves around the facet joint are cut or burned in order to provide pain relief. Critics of these procedures state that the nerve supply to other structures (e.g. ligaments and the small spinal muscles) is also affected; this may contribute to further facet joint instability and trauma.[19,20]

3) Patients with pain due to nerve root compression can receive a steroid injection into the space surrounding the spinal cord and nerve roots; this treatment is called an epidural injection. It decreases pain without significantly interfering with sensory or motor nerves. Advocates of epidural injections claim it provides immediate pain relief in 80 percent of patients;[25] the effects gradually dissolve over the following six months. One study, however, found no difference in pain relief between patients receiving an epidural injection and those who were injected with a placebo.[8] One risk of epidural injection is incorrect placement of the needle, which happens up to 25 percent of the time.[25] Serious complications include infections or inflammation of the meninges (the three outer coverings of the brain and spinal cord).[8]

4) Injection of a pain-killing substance with or without steroids can be used for diagnostic or therapeutic purposes in spinal or pelvic structures. If anesthetizing a facet joint provides dramatic relief, it identifies the site of the pain and may justify more extreme measures. The effects of a steroid injection may last months. However, over time repeated injections can destroy soft tissue.

Box 5-3

Key Points - Pain Inhibition

Inhibiting the perception of pain does not remove its causes, but it can provide significant relief to pain patients. Some treatments work by stimulating the production of endorphins, the body's own pain-killers. Others work by blocking pain at the spinal cord level through increased amounts of sensory stimulation. There are also medications and surgical procedures available when chronic pain levels are so high they interfere with an individual's ability to function.

Footnotes

1 *The Back Letter*, "Memo on Body Mechanics"
2 *The Back Letter*, Vol. 4, No. 6
3 Steven Brena, *Chronic Pain: America's Hidden Epidemic*
4 Rene Cailliet, *Low Back Pain Syndrome*
5 Annemarie Colbin, *Food and Healing*
6 Consumer Reports Books, *Health Quackery*
7 Pat Croce, "Put Stress to Rest"
8 John Cuckler, et al., "The Use of Epidural Steriods in the Treatment of Lumbar Radicular Pain"
9 Richard Deyo, et al., "A Controlled Trial of Transcutaneous Electrical Nerve Stimulation (TENS) and Exercise for Chronic Low Back Pain"
10 Richard DiFabio, "Clinical Assessment of Manipulation and Mobilization of the Lumbar Spine"
11 Neil Elgee, "Norman Cousins' Sick Laughter Redux"
12 Billy Glisan, et al., "Physiology of Active Exercise in Rehabilitation of Back Injuries"
13 David Imrie, *Goodbye Back Ache*
14 Kaplan & Tanner, *Musculoskeletal Pain and Disability*
15 Kessler & Hertling, *Management of Common Musculoskeletal Disorders*
16 Klein & Sobel, *Backache Relief*
17 David Lamb, "The Neurology of Spinal Pain"
18 G.D. Maitland, *Vertebral Manipulation*
19 Stanley Paris, "Anatomy as Related to Function and Pain"
20 Stanley Paris, "Physical Signs of Instability"
21 Stanley Paris, *The Spine*
22 *Physical Therapy Bulletin*, "Benefits of 'Humor Therapy' Promoted"
23 Richard Sternbach, *Pain Patients: Traits and Treatments*
24 Lynn Thomas, et al., "Physiological Work Performance in Chronic Low Back Disability"
25 Arthur White, "Injection Techniques for the Diagnosis and Treatment of Low Back Pain"
26 Judith Willis, "Back Pain: Ubiquitous, Controversial"

Chapter 6 -
Pain Management

Pain Clinics

"Pain and back centers have mushroomed since the 1970s. About 2,000 now exist. Because no two are alike and there are few follow-up studies, opinions vary about their effectiveness."
David Zinman[14]

Pain clinics are multidisciplinary centers offering a combination of physical therapy, occupational therapy, psychological testing, counseling, social work, pharmacology, vocational counseling, nursing and a variety of specializing physicians. Such clinics are effective because all the necessary treatment approaches are in one place at one time; fewer medical work-ups are needed and more options available. The major factor required is the patient's willing cooperation. Most people with chronic pain are said to have difficulties with drugs, dependence, depression, anxiety and/or physical deconditioning. The role of the clinic is to detoxify from drug use, to desensitize to pain perception, to provide relaxation training, basic exercises and physical conditioning and to teach patients to take an active role in managing their pain. The goal is not to cure, but to give patients the ability to live with their disabilities.

The philosophy of pain clinics varies; what governs the specific approach is most likely the director's specialty.[14] The different approaches used at the following four pain centers demonstrate this variation.

1) At the University of Miami center, chronic pain patients work through their pain; they are pushed to the limit, building up to rigorous physical training and exercise. The emphasis is on coping and functioning with the pain versus eliminating it.[14]

2) At Folsom Physical Therapy, the underlying premise is that pain causes no gain; the first step is to find the positions that cause pain and avoid them. The patient is then taught to be pain-free in all activities and learns to have control by being able to avoid painful positions.[12]

3) In the Casa Colina Program of Pain Management, the emotional/mental components of pain are recognized as crucial elements in the whole picture. The patient is expected to give up the invalid role and is taught assertiveness skills.[9]

4) A clinic in Stony Brook, New York, relies on a new machine which shows the precise degree of muscle exertion produced during exercise. It is used to monitor progress and to motivate patients to build muscle strength. It also supposedly provides evidence on whether a patient is exaggerating pain; a correlation is assumed between muscle exertion and pain production.[14]

A comprehensive pain program usually includes the following services:
- drug control or prescription
- rehabilitation specifically aimed at the disability
- posture and body mechanics
- exercises for strength and flexibility
- pacing instruction to teach appropriate rest/activity balance
- physical reconditioning
- relaxation techniques (biofeedback, hypnosis, visualization)
- modification of how pain is perceived
- pain inhibition (TENS, acupuncture)
- psychological counseling
- stress management
- assertiveness training
- vocational evaluation, counseling and rehabilitation
- nutrition

As is true of any therapeutic approach, pain clinics must individualize their programs to be successful. Pain clinics are highly rated by some experts because they provide diagnosis from a broad perspective and offer many different treatments. One author advises anyone with pain that lasts more than two months to contact a comprehensive pain clinic, but reports that only 3 percent of Americans with chronic pain do so.[5] However, another author reports that intensive programs for people with chronic pain may have only short-term success; one study showed that after six months, the results were only partly maintained.[3]

Pain Coping Skills

"There are disastrous side effects from pain because we focus on relief from a pain which usually has no clear cause and no clear cure; the real problem is not the pain, but how we handle it." Edward Abraham, MD[1]

Emotional factors, environmental reinforcement and secondary gains can perpetuate a patient's pain. (This is discussed in Chapter 3 under "Effects of Personality on Pain.") People can become victims to the pain, feeling trapped, threatened and unable to change.[10] The goal of pain management is to replace pain-perpetuating behaviors with new coping behaviors. Instead of waiting to take up life where it left off, patients are encouraged to make adjustments to their disabilities and to resume an active life. Pain management attempts to put the patient in charge. When a back problem becomes chronic, more and more responsibility for health care falls upon the person with pain. It is the patient who ultimately has the responsibility for coping with the pain, finding alternative employment, selecting the most appropriate treatment approaches and learning how to resume and maintain an active lifestyle.[2,4,13]

Practitioners have various strategies to help their chronic pain patients develop the inner resources necessary for successful pain management.

1) Reassure the patient that the pain is not malignant or life-threatening; address his concerns. The chances for successful coping are improved if the patient is not overly anxious.

2) Be frank and tell the patient that the condition is not likely to change; the pain will have to be endured.[13] Change the patient's focus from finding a cure to managing the pain.

3) Teach the patient to alter the way pain is perceived. When pain is controlling one's life, it is seen as a warning, a danger signal and a barrier to activity. Pain eventually becomes synonymous with movement. Patients can learn to discriminate between activity and pain; if they accept the pain as given, they can experience it while being active instead of having the same experience while being invalids.[1,4,10]

4) Help the patient develop self-reliance and coping skills; there are many treatment approaches that promote relaxation, confidence or a positive outlook.

5) Offer the patient specific guidelines for successful coping.
- Keep active and occupied.
- Direct yourself outward.
- Maintain a schedule compatible with the rest of the family and the world.
- Avoid advertising your suffering.
- Carry out an exercise routine suited to your needs.
- Commit yourself to a healthy lifestyle despite the hurt.
- Aim for the acceptance of pain without emotional distress.

Some pain experts have described chronic pain as a failure, including medicine's failure to adequately address acute pain and society's failure to encourage a personal commitment to healthy living. The patient also fails – in (1) meeting challenges, (2) maintaining dignity, (3) recognizing and dealing with negative feelings, and (4) exercising mental control over pain-producing impulses.[4] These practitioners believe that a mental turnaround is required of the patient before a physical turnaround is possible. In the treatment of chronic back pain therefore, it is up to the patient to acknowledge that the primary problem is emotional and that pain is an excuse to not get better.[1,7] Patients are taught that they have the responsibility for defusing their negative feelings and choosing to recover.[1]

Stress Reduction

"Warning: Aggravation Ahead" Highway Department Sign on Rte. 270 entering Washington D.C.

Relaxation techniques may be used to reduce muscle spasm or to stretch tight muscles. Other types of relaxation training reduce anxiety and improve a patient's sense of control; patients are encouraged to gain mental mastery over their tension. Many programs emphasize the importance of combining physical and mental relaxation. A partial list of the numerous methods used to promote relaxation follows.

- exercises
- physical conditioning
- progressive relaxation exercises (including Jacobson's)
- Alexander Technique
- dance therapy
- breathing exercises (including Fuch's and Jenck's)
- acupuncture and acupressure
- counseling
- meditation
- meditation on a single word or color (Benson's Technique or The Relaxation Response)
- behavior modification (receiving a reward for a desired physical response)
- energetics (combining body movements and verbalizations for the release of blocked energy and reintegration of mind and body)
- mental training exercises such as autogenic training (mental focusing on a short verbal phrase which suggests a state of physiological balance – "My arms and legs are warm." "My heartbeat is calm and regular.")
- visualization
- hypnosis or self-hypnosis
- biofeedback
- muscle inhibition techniques
- disciplines for mind and body (including yoga, Tai Chi and Zen)
- massage

Exercise is thought to reduce stress in two ways. As discussed in Chapter 5, activity stimulates the production of endorphins. Studies have indicated that high intensity exercise can raise pain tolerance, decrease pain sensation and elevate mood.[6] Another theory is that moderate exercise increases metabolism and uses up excess "catecholamines"; these are compounds produced by the body as a response to stress. Intense exercise, however, releases more catecholamines.[8]

Stress reduction techniques are also used to promote overall health or even to cure disease. Many alternative health practitioners emphasize the power of feelings to cause or cure health problems; individuals are encouraged to use their spiritual, mental and emotional strength and energy to improve their lives and health. Visualization, yoga, hypnosis, psychotherapy, meditation and relaxation training are examples of approaches used to teach patients to draw on their inner resources to direct positive energy toward the relief of back pain.

Researchers are deeply divided on the connection between attitude and disease. *"Twenty years ago, hardly anyone thought mind and body were related, but we have now swung to a belief just as simplistic and inaccurate that illness is created in the mind."* [11] The emphasis on personal responsibility can empower patients, but can also place an unfair burden on people with health problems. A positive outlook does help some patients feel better and certainly improves the quality of life, but it is not the cure for everyone's back pain.

Key Points - Pain Management

During an acute episode of back pain, practitioners attempt to pinpoint a diagnosis and find the treatment approach that will eliminate the pain and dysfunction. Treatment aimed specifically at chronic back pain has a different goal. Pain clinics, pain coping skills and stress reduction techniques are all used to help chronic pain patients successfully function with their disabilities.

Footnotes

1 Edward Abraham, *Freedom from Back Pain: An Orthopedist's Guide*
2 "Approaches to Musculoskeletal Problems" Symposium, Jane Derebery
3 *The Back Letter*, Vol. 4, No. 3
4 Steven Brena, *Chronic Pain: America's Hidden Epidemic*
5 Jean Carper, *Health Care, U.S.A.*
6 Pat Croce, "Put Stress to Rest"
7 Derebery & Tullis, "Delayed Recovery in the Patient with a Work Compensable Injury"
8 Billy Glisan, et al., "Physiology of Active Exercise in Rehabilitation of Back Injuries"
9 Harold Gottlieb, et al., "An Innovative Program for the Restoration of Patients with Chronic Back Pain"
10 Barbara Headley, "Pain Vs. Suffering"
11 Betsy Lehman, "Feeling Bad About Feeling Bad"

12   Edith Montgomery, "Folsom Physical Therapy – A Different Approach to Back
      Rehabilitation"
13   Richard Sternbach, *Pain Patients: Traits and Treatments*
14   David Zinman, "Focus on Back Pain"

Chapter 7 - Home Programs

" 'You'd best be getting home,' he said, 'The nights are very damp.'" Lewis Carroll, *Alice in Wonderland*

In their search for relief, most people with chronic pain visit numerous health practitioners and try numerous therapies. The hope is always there that the next one will be "the answer," correcting the underlying problem and removing the pain forever. When a treatment is unsuccessful in eliciting a cure, it is often abandoned. Others are continued indefinitely as if the underlying problem is still acute and should continue to be treated with acute measures. Some of the recommendations given to recently injured back pain patients have validity for the chronic pain patient; others do not.

Treatments Harmful When Overused

"The best things carried to excess are wrong." Charles Churchill, "The Rosciad"

There are approaches often recommended during the acute phase of back pain which are apt to be detrimental to the person with chronic pain. Their overuse can cause secondary problems or increase pain and dysfunction over time. These include prolonged or total bedrest, mechanical supports and pain-killing drugs.

Bedrest

Inactivity causes harmful systemic effects, a loss of calcium in the bones, delay of tissue healing, loss of muscle strength and psychological depression. Excessive bedrest for back pain has been proven to be not only useless, but detrimental.[3] Its well-known effects when prolonged may be a significant contributor to chronic disability in back patients.[12] Rest should always be interspersed with activity for those with chronic disabilities.

Braces, Corsets and Collars

Mechanical supports can immobilize a body part or correct poor align-ment. They are prescribed to transfer weight and movement away from the spine to other structures, increase abdominal support, decrease pressure on the disks, decrease use of spinal muscles for relief of spasm, increase patient awareness of correct posture or for a placebo effect where the use of a support gives the patient a sense of security. Braces, corsets and cervical collars should be used as a short-term solution; they should never be prescribed without a plan to eliminate them.[9,13] Total dependency on a brace allows the soft tissues of the spine to relinquish their supporting function so that the brace becomes the sole support; they interfere with normal movement of the spine and thereby potentially increase pain and dysfunction.

Medications

Certain medications can be helpful during acute episodes and others appropriate for people with chronic pain. However, back pain patients are advised to minimize drug use to avoid the dangers of side effects and physical or emotional addiction. Drug abuse is one of the most devastating complica-tions of chronic pain. People can become addicted to pain-killing or other medications; they may even use the pain to justify continued drug use instead of taking more positive measures.[2]

A possible exception is the use of anti-depressants for chronic pain;[1] this is discussed in Chapter 5 under "Medications."

Treatments Helpful to All

"Most back pain patients are best advised to live with their disorder and fight it with activity." Charles Fager, MD[5]

Treatment recommendations may be discontinued when total pain relief is not achieved, but some are beneficial to the whole person as well as the back and should be continued on a permanent basis. These include the incorporation of proper posture and body mechanics, an individualized physical conditioning program and attention to one's overall health needs.

Physical Conditioning

While excessive inactivity has been shown to have detrimental effects, exercise, in whatever form, is considered to have multiple benefits.
- promotion of cardiovascular fitness
- maintenance of muscle strength and endurance
- increase of blood flow to injured tissues
- elongation of soft tissues (muscles, tendons, joint capsules and ligaments)
- promotion of mental well-being
- reduction of stress
- pain inhibition

To optimize physical conditioning, "aerobic" exercises, such as walking, biking and swimming, should be selected. Aerobic exercises increase the body's use of oxygen and increase heart and lung activity through rhythmic, repetitive activities lasting over 20 minutes. Chronic back pain and its adjustments can cause a measurable reduction in physical fitness; this can be reversed in a short time with a simple, individualized activity program.[14] A program needs to be tailored so that it is appropriate to each person's specific disability level.

Posture and Body Mechanics

Poor use of the back is considered a possible cause or contributing factor in virtually every type of back pain; poor posture stresses the joints, disks and soft tissues of the spine. No treatment can undo the harmful effects of continual misuse of the back, but it is never too late to learn how to stand, sit, bend, lift and sleep correctly. For many years, flattening the lumbar curve through the "pelvic tilt routine" was considered the appropriate approach for protecting the back. Most specialists now advocate maintenance of the natural, gentle curves of neck and back during all activities. In addition, changing position frequently is recommended, whatever the activity, to unload joints, relax muscles and redistribute pressure on weight-bearing surfaces.

There are excellent guides for posture and body mechanics for people with all levels of back pain; they should be read and applied so that the spine won't continue to be subjected to repeated injury and stress through improper use. (See "Recommended Reading" at the end of Chapter 8.)

Treatments Helpful to Some

"People talk fundamentals and superlatives and then make some changes of detail." Oliver Wendell Holmes

There are some acute treatments which provide significant help to certain people with chronic back pain; these same treatments may have no affect on other individuals. They include a program of specific back exercises, the use of heat or ice, the use of seating or positioning equipment and special diets.

Back Exercises

Physical conditioning seems to benefit all kinds of back problems, but there is insufficient information regarding the effects of specific exercises on back pain.[8] No support exists for the use of preprinted hand-outs which assume every patient requires the same exercise routine; exercise programs must be individualized. Exercises can be prescribed to increase flexibility, strength and/or endurance; flexion exercises benefit some patients, extension exercises others and many people should address both of these muscle groups for balanced strength. Exercises which emphasize movement reeducation promote motor "skill"; back pain causes overuse, disuse or misuse of certain muscles, disrupting normal postural balance and movement patterns.[6,7] Whatever the specific type of routine recommended, many people with back pain feel they are significantly improved if they stick to an individualized exercise program.

Heat and Ice

During a particularly painful episode or a relapse, heat is often helpful for the reduction of muscle spasm. Ice, however, is the recommended treatment when inflammation is present; two to three minute ice massages are thought to be more effective than an ice pack.[1]

Equipment

Prescription and non-prescription equipment is available to help people maintain a proper position. Sitting for prolonged periods is often difficult for people with chronic back pain; adjustable office chairs which encourage an upright posture, lumbar or cervical rolls to maintain the curves of the back, and thoracic or sacral supports to stabilize the spine are all examples of positioning equipment that may help with pain control. Such devices, however, are no substitute for learning proper posture and body mechanics and frequent changes of position.

Diet

An improper diet and lifestyle is thought by some to be the root of most medical problems, while a natural foods diet based on whole grains and vegetables is the necessary foundation of health and well-being.[10] One author states, *"Fifty percent of spinal pain can result from red meats."*[11] Some diets and vitamin therapies claim to shrink bone spurs, restore joint flexibility and alleviate low back pain; the elimination of meat, milk and nightshades (potatoes, tomatoes, tobacco) is frequently advocated.[5]

Key Points - Home Programs

Some of the treatment approaches used for back pain patients are inappropriate for the person with chronic pain and can even contribute to physical and/or emotional dysfunction if continued beyond the acute phase. Other treatments, while not eliminating back pain, are helpful when continued indefinitely on a regular basis. Individuals have to find their own unique combination of therapies and lifestyle adaptations which will minimize pain and promote overall health.

Footnotes

1 *The Back Letter*, Vol. 4, No. 6
2 Steven Brena, *Chronic Pain: America's Hidden Epidemic*
3 Rene Cailliet, *Low Back Pain Syndrome*
4 Annemarie Colbin, *Food and Healing*

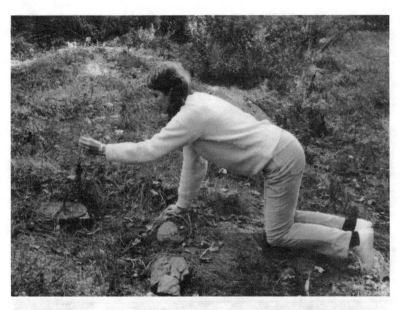

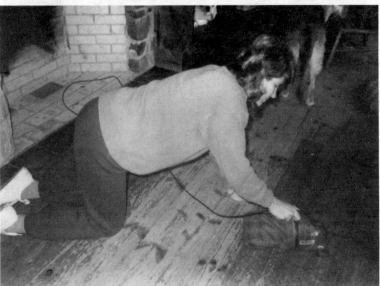

If stooping or squatting down is a problem, a variety of indoor and outdoor tasks, such as gardening and vacuuming, can be done in an all - fours or kneeling position.

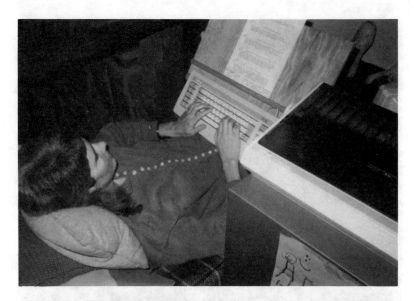

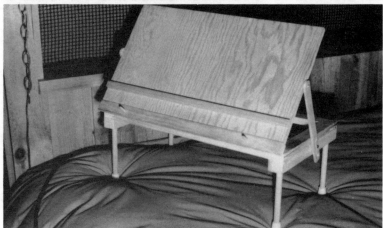

A made - to - order "supine desk" can be used for any lying down activity. Having an efficient work surface when you are lying down means you can be busy and productive while resting your back. You can even play a musical instrument! (see opposite page) The desk pictured was designed to use with a computer; the keyboard hangs from the pegs in front and a ridge holds papers. (Plans for this supine desk are available; send $3.00 and a self - addressed, stamped, legal - sized envelope to Roy Lawrence, 20 Park St., Bath, Maine 04530.)

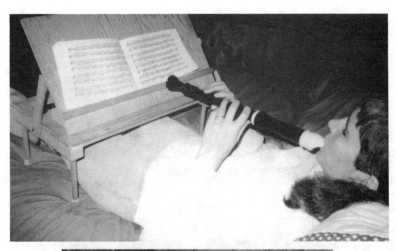

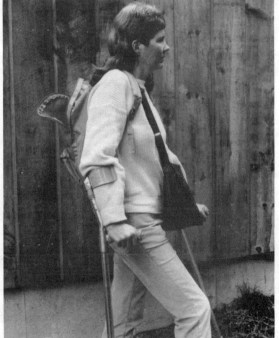

Certain pieces of equipment can make community activities easier on the back. For shopping trips or sightseeing, a bag with a long carrying strap, a knapsack and crutches are aides which maximize independence and comfort.

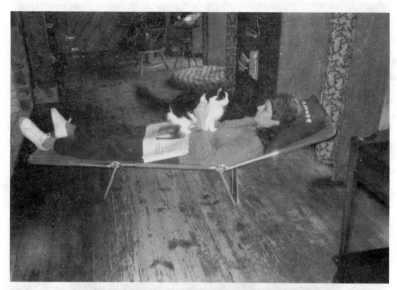

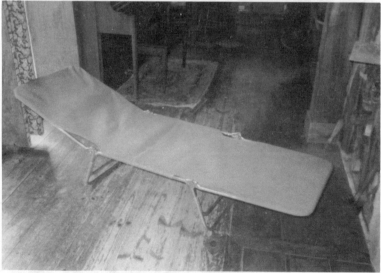

If you need to lie down frequently, a portable lounge chair can be used for working or socializing at home or out in public. Put an adjustable strap on it and you're ready for any occasion! (see opposite page) This model is available from L.L. Bean's in Freeport, Maine; it weighs only 9 pounds.

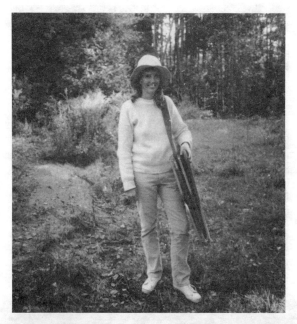

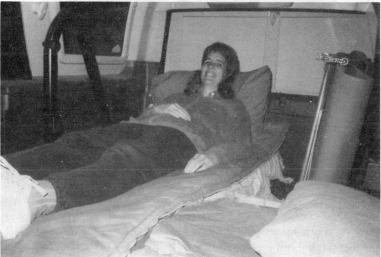

For traveling long distances, a car bed which allows you to see out the front windshield lets you ride confortably, share the sights with the person driving and arrive at your destinatiuon refreshed. The vehicle pictured is a Toyota 4 - Runner with a 6" piece of foam in the back.

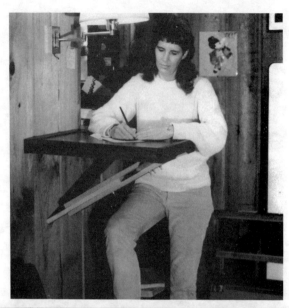

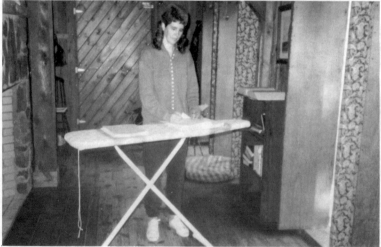

Build or create a standing desk, if prolonged sitting is impossible. A stand - up table can be hinged to a wall and dropped when not in use. An adjustable ironing board makes an excellent work surface for standing activities.

Photography by Frederick Valente

Chapter 8 - Self-Help

"Human felicity is produced not so much by great pieces of good fortune that seldom happen, as by little advantages that occur every day." Benjamin Franklin

Perhaps the first step in the management of chronic back pain is to be allowed to have and express the feelings of guilt, sadness, frustration or anger which accompany this condition. But when an acute backache turns into a chronic disability, there comes a time to stop comparing life-as-it-is to life-as-it-was. It is hard to move forward while continuing to wait for the pain to go away.

After all the treatments espoused by traditional and alternative health practitioners have been tried, people with chronic back pain have to discover for themselves the many ways that make managing back pain easier. This chapter offers strategies . . .

1) to maximize one's physical resources in order to lead an active life without an excessive level of pain, and

2) for coping emotionally in order to accept and make the most of one's new life.

Chapter 8

Maximizing Your Physical Resources

"Self-love, my liege, is not so vile a sin, as self-neglecting." Shakespeare, *King Henry V*,
Act 2, Scene 4

There are many ways for the person with chronic back pain to make job,
home, travel and socializing more comfortable. Creativity in making adaptations is required; determine what you want to do, then set about discovering
how to make it possible or easier. Some things may only be accomplished
to your satisfaction by gritting your teeth and ignoring the pain, but these
should be kept to a minimum. Consistently overstepping your physical limits
eventually pushes your coping skills to the point of collapse. Your long-term
goal is to achieve the highest possible level of activity at which you can
maintain emotional stability. Specific suggestions for reaching that goal
follow.

Changes in Lifestyle

Changing the way you perform activities, instead of eliminating them
altogether, can decrease back pain significantly. Certain tasks, however,
may be too strenuous to undertake; when you determine the lifestyle
changes that work for you, stick to them and also make them clear to
friends and family.

1) Find the right balance between activity and relaxation. Make both rest
periods and a daily exercise program priorities. Stop yourself when it's time
to rest; get used to leaving a job undone until your next "up time". Don't put
off the exercise either; you'll pay for the inconsistency with more pain and
less accomplished in the long run.

2) Change position regularly, whether resting, working or traveling.
Learn proper body mechanics and make them a part of your everyday life.
(See "Recommended Reading" at the conclusion of this chapter for books
which promote correct use of the back.)

3) Plan ahead so you can fit what you want to get done into your normal
"up time." When you're having a bad week, listen to your body and adjust
your activities accordingly.

4) Do as much as you can independently, using whatever adaptations are
necessary, but when appropriate ask for help. People are usually happy to
be of assistance, but don't always know when to offer.

5) Hire a person to help clean the house; yes, it is a luxury, but the alternative is to use your valuable and limited resources in housekeeping when you could be doing something more rewarding. This also applies to mowing the lawn, changing the oil in the car, repairing the screen door, etc. An alternative is to reassign household chores so that other members of the family take over the most physically stressful tasks.

6) Use common sense when purchasing clothes; footwear should definitely be friendly to the back. Avoid clothes that are a struggle to put on or that sacrifice mobility and comfort for style. Arrange your wardrobe to minimize bending and twisting by putting the most used items in top drawers or in the front of the closet.

7) Arrange your kitchen and workroom to avoid taking heavy items out of low places. Make sure your work surface is high enough and close enough for you to do kitchen and household chores comfortably while either standing or sitting.

8) Supermarket employees are usually very nice about not only putting your groceries in the car, but also unloading the cart at the register or getting a heavy item off the shelf. You may want to buy large items in easy-to-lift smaller sizes, or you can leave the non-perishables in the car until another family member can help unload and put them away.

Equipment
Some adaptations are expensive, but it is hard to put a price on an aid that can increase comfort and efficiency. Using special equipment in public requires putting comfort above the opinions of other people.

9) Do whatever it takes to make the bed, couch, chair or work station where you spend the most time comfortable. Use whatever combination of pillows, cushions, cervical or lumbar rolls is necessary to ensure that your back is positioned correctly at home, at work and even while socializing. Buy extra pillows to keep at work or in the car to avoid lugging equipment or forgetting to bring it. Inflatable or roll-up travel pillows are available commercially to cut down on the bulk. This paraphernalia may be cumbersome and look unusual, but you'll be able to fully enjoy your outings and be more efficient in your work if you're positioned comfortably. You'll be better company too.

10) If sitting is a problem, build, buy or find a high enough surface to be used as a standing-up desk. An adjustable ironing board can make an

excellent work surface; it should be high enough for you to work efficiently without leaning over.

11) If you require periods of lying down throughout the day, have a "supine desk" built to meet your specifications; this permits you to be active while resting and to know that the down time is not wasted. Supine desks can be modified specifically for writing, reading or computers.

12) Buy a cordless telephone to avoid getting up repeatedly when you're trying to rest your back.

13) Buy a hand vacuum; nothing is worse for a back than vacuuming and a mini-vac lets you handle the minor disasters. It can be used from a hands and knees position if squatting down is difficult.

14) If you work lying down, use light-weight books, pens that write without the help of gravity and clipboards to hold your papers; they will help you avoid awkward positions when resting.

15) Once you have found a chair that is comfortable for your back, you can take it along with you while out in public. Unfortunately, this requires carrying a piece of furniture which may be neither light-weight nor easily portable, but it will be worth it for activities requiring prolonged sitting. If someone offers to carry it, say yes.

16) Portable lounge chairs can be used to lie down at work, meetings, theaters, picnics, church – just about anywhere. Their disadvantage is that you may feel like an invalid, lying down in public. Their significant advantage is that you can participate in any activity without increasing your pain, as long as you can find the room to open up the chair. (Durable light-weight [9 lb.] lounge chairs are available from L.L. Bean in Freeport, Maine for approximately $60. 1-800-221-4221.)

17) The overuse of crutches can change your posture and weaken muscles, and you may feel they would make you look more handicapped than you are. However, there are times when crutches are an invaluable aid, allowing people with certain types of back problems to participate at a level they couldn't otherwise achieve. Crutches take some weight off the spine and can significantly increase your up time. They are especially useful for shopping sprees, standing-around social activities and visiting tourist spots such as museums. With crutches you may look disabled, but you can feel better and last longer during a special outing.

18) When using crutches or carrying equipment, it is helpful to have a pocketbook or tote bag with a long strap that can be put over your head.

Backpacks are also very useful for shopping. These items keep the weight of their contents near the center of your body and leave your hands free.

Traveling

Traveling is especially hard on backs, with the bumps, vibrations and long periods in one position. The physical stress of traveling can prevent you from being at your best when you arrive at your destination.

19) Features that make a car more comfortable to ride in or drive include automatic transmission, power steering, hand brake, reclining adjustable front seats, adjustable steering wheel, sufficient leg room and easy-to-open trunk. A cervical collar, lumbar roll or sacral support may be helpful when driving to keep the neck and low back positioned correctly during the ride. A car that can accommodate a bed gives a whole new dimension to traveling. You can relieve the driver for short periods and still arrive at your destination refreshed rather than in agony. It is especially convenient to have a bed that can face forward, allowing you a view out the front windshield and cutting down on motion sickness. (One vehicle that can accommodate such a bed is the Toyota 4-Runner, without the optional rear seats.)

20) Airplane seats recline, but only about 30 degrees. First-class tickets are expensive, but the leg room and increased recline of the seats could make a difference in how well you can function on your vacation or business trip. Overseas flights are usually the only ones with fully reclining seats. If prolonged standing or sitting is a problem, ask the airline for wheelchair assistance; the brief time spent sitting in the wheelchair may be preferable to the long walk to the terminal and the long wait for your luggage. You can pack an inflatable air mattress in your suitcase to use as a bed in a rental station wagon.

Maximizing Your Emotional Resources

"The cure for anything is salt water – sweat, tears or the sea." Isak Dinesen

In addition to discovering the adaptations that help your body, you have to hone your coping skills in order to manage the emotional offshoots of chronic back pain. Physically you have to find the balance between rest and activity; emotionally you have to allow yourself to vent your feelings without letting pain consume your thoughts. You cannot sustain the same level of

Chapter 8

focus on your health that was appropriate during the acute onset of pain; self-esteem and satisfaction mustn't be based on the things you can no longer do. The goal of a person with chronic back pain is to say "I'm fine!" and mean it. What follows are suggestions to help in the struggle to be fine.

1) Be open to new approaches, but don't get sucked in by extravagant claims or someone else's success. Learn about various treatments; if they feel right for you and are administered by legitimate practitioners with a good track record, give them a try. Don't think you have to try them all; friends may say, "What have you got to lose?" and the answer is time, money, false hopes, self-esteem, side-effects and being in limbo while you wait for the results. Feel free, too, to take from a treatment the part that works for you; you don't have to adopt a whole new philosophy of life to gain something from an approach.

2) When the time is right, allow yourself to let go of the search for answers and cures; the energy spent on the search can be used instead to manage the pain and resume an active life.

3) Allow yourself to grieve your losses; you will find new goals and rewards, but you have lost a part of your life and you have a right to be sad about that. People with chronic disabilities go through the stages of grieving common to those with terminal illnesses, (denial, anger, grief, acceptance). The process may be repeated again and again, especially with a relapse or increased level of dysfunction.

4) Learn to accept help; if you have always taken pride in your self-sufficiency, it is a humbling experience to suddenly need other people for emotional and physical support. Remember that if they were in pain, you would be glad to have a way to help them and be flattered to be asked.

5) Develop a new definition of your baseline and what "fine" means to you. If you compare yourself to how you used to be, you will never be fine.

6) Don't worry about what acquaintances think of your adaptations or your choices. You're the one living with your pain and your decisions. Others may think you could be doing better; what's important is how you feel. Recognize that comments which strike you as insensitive are probably intended to help.

7) Recognize that each plan for coping with pain must be tailormade; no one form of pain control works for everyone and all the advice you get should be examined with a critical eye. You're the only one who can select the best overall plan for yourself.

8) Although you may feel totally unequipped to do so, you must now be in charge of your health care. Others can provide information and support, but the responsibility for fact finding, understanding the meaning and consequences of pain, seeking help, creating breakthroughs and developing a new way of life is yours.

9) As time goes by, you will learn what to do and not to do to hold your pain at manageable levels. However, don't drive yourself crazy trying to figure out your physical ups and downs; you can adapt your lifestyle to control the pain level, but your back will have cycles that seem to bear no relation to anything you have done. Try to enjoy the good periods without worrying how long they'll last; think of the bad ones as just part of the cycle.

10) Regardless of the amount of rest time you require, don't consider yourself an invalid. Get dressed in the morning; lie on top of the bed instead of in the bed; accomplish something every day (writing a letter, mending a shirt, paying the bills); take over a family job you can do (keeping the checkbook, making business calls, planning menus); plan something to look forward to every day (a new book, a friend for lunch, a favorite radio show). You will feel less disabled and have something positive to share with your family.

11) Avoid blaming others or outside circumstances for your pain. Feeling like a helpless victim only leads to bitterness and isolation. Seek professional help for the psychological offshoots of pain if they are interfering with your ability to function. If the negative feelings are long-lasting and overwhelming, it is a smart and positive step to get counseling to learn how to manage them; it doesn't mean the pain is in your head.

12) Recognize that the people close to you, especially your spouse or partner, have suffered losses of their own. Their lives have changed too and they may not feel justified in expressing their own fears and sadness because they are not the ones suffering physical pain. Problems and events continue to happen in their lives and they also need time to share.

13) Back pain may make sexual relations difficult, but the pleasure and comfort of physical intimacy is as important to you and your partner as ever. Find ways to continue to be sexually active with a minimum of back pain; books such as Lauren Hebert's *Sex and Back Pain* can help.

14) Allow yourself a chance to occasionally voice your frustrations over the changes that chronic back pain has brought to your life. Anger or depression will crop up from time to time; telling someone about it helps

diffuse the feelings so you can carry on again. Find a friend or support group who can relate to your situation and with whom you can share. You can gripe about your limitations, listen to your friend's complaints and know that someone truly understands.

15) Books about people with disabilities can validate your feelings and let you know you're not alone; many are moving and inspiring. But avoid chronicles of the heroes and martyrs who accomplish miracles; they can set you up for feeling inadequate and guilty.

16) Find something you love to do and can be committed to; it keeps you going and helps you focus outside the pain. Service work is important; volunteers are needed at all skill levels and you will know you are still a contributing member of society.

17) Choose what is most important for you to do during the upcoming week and plan ahead to ensure that you can accomplish it without excessive pain. However, special occasions may merit overdoing it and paying the price the next day; if you can cherish the memories and satisfaction for months to come, the physical set-back may be worth it. It feels good to have that choice. Often you can get away with one overindulgence if you don't make a habit of pushing your limits.

18) Since back pain can limit every part of your life, you may feel that you have had to give up everything. Consider instead that you may have to do things differently, more slowly, with adaptive aids, less often or in a different position. Don't eliminate the things you love to do before using your ingenuity, and that of your friends and family, to find ways to make them possible. If you were a jogger, become a walker; if you were a gardener, weed on hands and knees for short periods or put your plants in a container at standing height; if you can no longer perform your job, cut the hours, adapt the workplace or explore a whole new career. Be proud of your past accomplishments, not bitter because they're over; new accomplishments are yet to come.

19) Don't let anyone blame you for your pain; do your best to find and incorporate the methods that minimize it and live your life with as positive an approach as possible. Nurture your sense of humor. Give yourself credit for how well you manage!

20) The day will come when you realize you have a life again – your pain is no longer the center of the universe. You're even in a position to help others who are struggling to manage their back pain. By listening and sharing

what you have learned, you'll discover how far you've come and how much you have to offer.

Recommended Reading

Lauren Hebert, *Sex and Back Pain* (a practical guide for finding comfortable positions for sex)

Barbara Headley, *Chronic Pain: Life Out of Balance* (an easy-to-read booklet on chronic pain issues with cartoon drawings)

Klein & Sobel, *Backache Relief* (the results of a large survey of back pain patients)

Robin McKenzie, *Treat Your Own Back* (a guide to causes of back pain and specific exercise programs)

Melnick, Saunders & Saunders, *Managing Back Pain* (an easy-to-understand explanation of the effects of posture on the back, with recommended exercises)

Sefra Pitzele, *We Are Not Alone* (a book that explores the difficulties of living with chronic illness and offers practical help)

Cheri Register, *Living With Chronic Illness* (another personal view of chronic illness. Both Pitzele and Register are very helpful from an emotional standpoint.)

Duane Saunders, *The Back Care Program* (a practical and inexpensive guide for proper posture in all kinds of activities – a must!)

Duane Saunders, *For Your Neck* (a booklet on the effects of posture on neck pain, with recommended exercises)

Julie Zimmerman, *The Almanac of Back Pain Treatments* (an in-depth examination of the entire range of traditional and alternative treatment approaches for back pain, including their pros and cons)

Julie Zimmerman, *The Diagnosis and Misdiagnosis of Back Pain* (an in-depth examination of the processes used to diagnose back pain, the approaches of different health professionals and the conditions which cause back pain)

Key Points - Self-Help

Back pain restricts normal activities at home, at work and in social situations; ignoring the pain is too emotionally demanding in the long run to be an effective solution. People who live with back problems have to allow themselves to accept, even seek out, the physical and emotional support they need. They have to take charge of their lives, finding ways to be active and having confidence in their decisions. This chapter offers 20 suggestions to help individuals with chronic back pain lead active lives without excessive pain levels, and 20 suggestions to help them take the necessary steps to be both supported and independent.

Conclusion: Moving On

Chronic Back Pain: Moving On presents the opinions, both professional and personal, concerning chronic back problems. It covers the range of management options for people with this disability. It attempts to give you, the person living with back pain, enough information to understand the effects of chronic pain on your life and the treatment and self-help possibilities that are available to you. The goal is to allow you to make informed decisions to help in the difficult task of finding the answers that will minimize your back pain. When you have explored your options and followed through on your choices, then relegate the pain to a less central place in your life. It's time to return to the essential task of making the best of your world and yourself!

Appendix A

Glossary

abduction - movement away from the midline of the body

active - performed through the effort of muscle contraction following nerve stimulation

acupressure - treatment approach using deep thumb or finger pressure on acupuncture points

acupuncture - treatment approach using needles inserted into the skin at points representing the body's meridians

acute - of recent onset; having a short, relatively severe course

acutherapy - acupuncture or acupressure

adduction - movement toward the midline of the body

adhesion - abnormal binding down of soft tissue

aerobics - exercise that increases the body's use of oxygen

ambulation - walking

ankylosing spondylitis - a form of arthritis, also called Marie Strumpel's disease

annulus fibrosis - the outer part of an intervertebral disk

anomaly - abnormality

antagonist - the muscle which performs movement in the opposite direction to the muscle being discussed

anterior - toward the front of the body

anterior dysfunction - displacement of the sacrum relative to the ilia, occurring on forward flexion

anterior superior iliac spine - bony landmark on the pelvis commonly called the "hip bone"

anterolateral - angled toward the front and side of the body

arachnoid - the middle of the three meninges

arthritis - a condition characterized by inflammation of the joints

articular - pertaining to a joint

articular cartilage - cartilaginous surface of a joint at the end of a bone

articular process - superior or inferior bony prominence of a vertebra which forms a facet joint with an adjacent vertebra

ASIS - see anterior superior iliac spine

asymptomatic - without symptoms; painless

atrophy - wasting or shrinking of muscle fibers

auto-immune - pertaining to conditions in which the body produces antibodies against its own tissues

autonomic nervous system - portion of the nervous system concerned with regulation of the heart muscle, smooth muscle and glands

back muscles - see spinal muscles

back school - a class offered by PT departments which teaches proper use of the spine

bedrest, total - bedrest during which any weight-bearing is eliminated or minimized

bilateral - involving both right and left sides of the body

biofeedback - a modality which visually or auditorally represents physiological responses of the body to enable patients to learn to consciously produce physical changes

body mechanics - the posture of the body in motion

bone - hard, immobile structure which makes up the skeleton or framework of the body

bone scan - radiographic test involving the injection of dye into a vein in order to identify diseases of bone

bone spur - abnormal growth of bony tissue often associated with degenerative changes

capsule - see joint capsule

cartilage - hard, structural tissue which makes up part of the skeleton; found at the ends of bones, ribs and joint surfaces

CAT scan - computerized axial tomography; a radiographic test which provides a three-dimensional picture of bone and soft tissue

catecholamines - compounds produced by the body in response to stress

cauda equina syndrome - a serious condition in which a nerve or nerves in the lower part of the spinal canal are compressed, causing bladder symptoms

central nervous system - the brain and spinal cord

cerebro-spinal fluid - a fluid produced by the brain which is contained between the meninges and which serves a shock-absorbing role for the central nervous system

cervical - pertaining to the neck region

cervical roll - cylindrical pillow placed behind the neck to maintain the cervical lordosis

chronic - long-lasting; pertaining to a medical condition lasting longer than three to six months

chronic pain syndrome - long-term pain which is reinforced by the environment and associated with a specific personality profile

coccyx - the vertebral segments comprising the tailbone

contract - shorten, referring to a muscle when stimulated

contraction - tensing or shortening of a muscle in response to a nerve stimulus

contraindicated - to be avoided; not recommended

contralateral - pertaining to the opposite side of the body

cortical bone - outer part of the shaft of a bone

cortisone - a hormone with anti-inflammatory properties

counterstrain - a technique which maintains the muscle in a relaxed, non-strained posture for 90 seconds

cranial - pertaining to the skull or head

craniosacral rhythm - the pulse produced by the cyclical production of CSF

CSF - see cerebro-spinal fluid

CT scan - see CAT scan

deafferation - the cutting of a sensory nerve

dermatome - skin area innervated by one spinal nerve

diathermy - machine which uses electricity to apply heat to surface tissues

differential diagnosis - the process of ruling out possible pathology to arrive at a definitive diagnosis

disc - see disk

disk - the structure located between the vertebral bodies, composed of a fibrous outer ring and an inner gelatin-like center

diskectomy - a surgical procedure to remove the disk or nucleus of the disk

disk fragment - extruded piece of the nucleus of the disk

diskography - a radiographic procedure in which dye is injected into a disk to identify a rupture

dislocation - total disruption of the opposing surfaces of a joint

DO - doctor of osteopathy

dural sheath (dura) - the outer covering of a nerve root

dura mater (dura) - the outermost of the three meninges which covers the brain and spinal cord
dysfunction - increased, decreased or abnormal movement

electromyography - diagnostic test in which needle electrodes inserted into muscle tissue relay
    electrical impulses from the muscle in order to identify nervous system diseases
electrotherapy - the therapeutic use of electricity
embryological - formed during the development of a fetus
EMG - see electromyography
endorphin - natural pain-killing substance produced by the body
endurance - lasting power; ability to maintain a position or perform numerous repetitions of a
    movement
ER - external rotation
erector spinae - back muscles which extend the trunk
ergonomics - adaptation of the workplace and equipment to accommodate an injured worker
extensibility - amount of stretch in a tissue
extension - motion of straightening a joint or body part
extensor muscles - see spinal muscles
external rotation - hip or shoulder movement in which the long bone of the thigh or arm rolls
    outward
extrusion - escaping of tissue outside its normal boundaries

facet joint - a synovial joint formed by the articular processes of two vertebrae
facilitation - see muscle facilitation
fascia - connective tissue of the body
femur - thigh bone
fiber - small segment of connective or muscle tissue; a nerve process
fibrillation - spontaneous contractions of individual muscle cells or fibers
fibromyalgia - see fibrositis
fibromyositis - see fibrositis
fibrositis - a condition characterized by diffuse tender areas of musculoskeletal tissues
flexion - motion of bending a joint or body part
function - use; movement
functional mobility - ability of the body to move normally to perform activities of daily living
functional restoration - work hardening
fusion - a surgical procedure in which bone fragments are inserted into an unstable joint to form
    a solid mass of bone

gate control theory - concept that pain sensations are blocked at the spinal cord by sensory
    stimulation
golfer's lift - stance incorporating extension of the non-weight bearing leg when bending forward
GP - general practitioner
gluteals - muscles at the back and sides of the pelvis which extend or abduct the hip
gluteal sets - tensing of the gluteus maximus muscles by squeezing the buttocks together

hamstrings - the muscles at the back of the thigh which extend the hip and flex the knee
herniated, herniation - see ruptured, rupture
holism - approach to health care which emphasizes the whole person
hyperextension - extension past a neutral trunk position
hypermobility - excessive movement of joints

hypomobility - below-average movement of joints
hypertonus - excessive amount of muscle tone

iatrogenic - caused by medical treatment
iliac crest - large curved portion of the upper pelvis, starting at what is commonly called the "hip bone"
ilium (pl. - ilia) - part of the pelvis which lies posterior and superior and forms a joint with the
    sacrum
impingement - compression, usually referring to a nerve root compression due to a disk rupture
inhibition - see muscle inhibition
innervation - nerve supply to a body part, usually referring to the nerve which stimulates a
    specific muscle
inominates - the joint surfaces of the pelvis which connect with the sacrum
internal rotation - a motion of the shoulder or hip joint in which the long bone of the upper arm
    or thigh rolls inward
interspinous ligaments - short ligaments connecting spinous processes of the vertebrae
intra-abdominal pressure - the tension of the contents of the abdomen against a contraction of
    the abdominal muscles
IR - internal rotation
internship - the year of hospital training following medical school
intervertebral - between the vertebrae
ischemia - decreased blood supply
ischium - part of the pelvis which lies posterior and inferior
isometrics - muscle contractions in which no joint movement occurs

joint - moveable part of the body's skeleton where the ends of two bones are joined
joint capsule - the sheath which surrounds and protects a synovial joint
joint play - small, involuntary movements in a joint in response to an outside force

kinesiology - the applied study of the principles and mechanics of movement
kinesiotherapy - a profession providing rehabilitation under the direction of physiatrist
KT - kinesiotherapist
kyphosis - convex curve of the spine, normal in the thoracic and sacral areas

lamina - the posterior part of the vertebral arch
laminectomy - surgical removal of the posterior arch of a vertebra, usually done to relieve nerve
    root compression from a ruptured disk
lateral flexion - movement of the neck or trunk to the side, away from the body's midline
lengthening contraction - tensing of a muscle to control movement in a direction opposite to its
    normal action
lesion - site of an injury
ligament - tough inelastic tissue which supports joints
longitudinal ligaments - long anterior and posterior ligaments running the length of the spinal
    column and connecting the vertebral bodies
long-sitting - sitting position with hips flexed and knees extended
lordosis - concave curve of the spine, normal in the cervical and lumbar areas
low back syndrome - vague diagnosis referring to non life-threatening conditions affecting the
    lumbo-sacral spine and its related structures
lumbago - common term for backache
lumbar - pertaining to the low back area

lumbar roll - approximately four-inch cylindrical pillow used to maintain a lumbar lordosis

magnetic resonance imaging - a non-invasive diagnostic test in which magnetic waves are used to image soft tissues

malingering - pretending to be ill

malleolus - ankle bone

manipulation - treatment approach in which the practitioner imparts a sudden thrust to realign body structures and/or reduce functional limitations

manual therapy - treatment in which the practitioner's hands are used to effect changes in the body

MD - medical doctor; one who has graduated from a four-year medical school

meninges - the three membranes which surround the brain and spinal cord

meniscus - crescent-shaped structure made up of cartilage and fibrous tissue which attaches to a joint capsule and extends into a joint

MENS - microcurrent therapy

meridian - one of 12 channels of vital energy in the body; a concept used in acupuncture

microcurrent therapy - form of electrotherapy which uses a current of low amperage to promote healing

mixers - chiropractors who use other treatment forms in addition to manipulation

mobilization - gentle form of manual therapy used to restore normal movement to body structures

MRI - magnetic resonance imaging

muscle - structure made up of elastic, contractile fibers which shortens when stimulated by a nerve to produce movement at a joint

muscle energy techniques - treatment which uses nervous system mechanisms to inhibit or facilitate a specific muscle

muscle facilitation - technique which uses nervous system mechanisms to increase muscle tone and stimulate a muscle to contract

muscle fatigue - technique using a strong contraction of a tight muscle to cause subsequent inhibition and relaxation of that muscle

muscle inhibition - use of nervous system mechanisms to reduce tone or spasm in tight muscles

muscle tone - see tone

myelogram - a radiographic test in which cerebro-spinal fluid is removed from the space sur rounding the spinal cord and dye is injected in order to identify nerve root compression

myofascial - pertaining to the muscles and their surrounding connective tissue

myofascial pain syndrome - see fibrositis

nerve - a cell which transmits impulses within the nervous system to carry information to and from the brain or spinal cord; a bundle of nerve projections and their coverings

nerve root - part of the nervous system connecting the spinal cord and peripheral nerves which lies within the spinal canal

nerve root compression - pressure against a nerve root, commonly from a ruptured disk or bone spur, which produces pain and neurologic signs

neurological - neurologic

neurologic signs - symptoms which indicate involvement of the nervous system; with nerve root compression, numbness, weakness, decreased reflexes

neurology - a medical specialty which treats diseases of the nervous system

neurosurgery - a medical specialty where operations are performed on the nervous system or its surrounding structures

nightshades - a category of foods which includes potatoes, tomatoes and tobacco

NMR - nuclear magnetic resonance (see MRI)
nociceptive - painful, injury producing
nucleus pulposis - the gelatin-like, water-binding center of an intervertebral disk

obliques - the two abdominal muscles which perform diagonal trunk flexion
occupational therapy - an allied medical profession concerned with functional activities for rehabilitation, developmental and psychiatric treatment
opposition - state in which body surfaces are in close proximity and parallel to each other, as with joint surfaces or thumb to finger pad
organic - physical; pertaining to the body
orthopedic - pertaining to the musculoskeletal system
orthopedic surgeon - an MD specializing in operations to correct conditions of the musculos-keletal system
orthopod - slang for orthopedic surgeon
osteoarthritis - condition characterized by localized degenerative changes in joints
osteophyte - bone spur
osteoporosis - abnormal thinning of the bones
osteopath - a graduate from a four-year school of osteopathic medicine with a DO degree
OT - occupational therapist or occupational therapy

pain behavior - actions and personality characteristics typical of patients whose chronic pain is reinforced by their environments
pain clinic - a rehabilitation center with a multidisciplinary approach to chronic pain
pain coping - therapeutic techniques to help chronic pain patients adjust to their disabilities
pain inhibition - techniques used to block the transmission of pain messages to the brain
pain management - therapeutic techniques to help chronic pain patients minimize their pain and maximize their function
palpation - examination by touch
paraspinal - in the area of the spine
paraspinal muscles - see spinal muscles
parasympathetic nervous system - the cranio-sacral portion of the autonomic nervous system
paravertebral - in the area of the vertebrae
paravertebral muscles - see spinal muscles
paresthesia - abnormal sensation, including pins-and-needles, tingling, burning
passive - performed by an outside force without active muscle contraction
pathology - diseased or abnormal state
pedicle - segment of the vertebral arch which joins the vertebral body to the lamina
pelvic obliquity - asymmetry of the pelvic ring creating a wind-blown effect
pelvic tilt - upward movement of the front of the pelvis which flattens the lumbar curve and which is accomplished by a contraction of the abdominal and gluteal muscles
pelvis - large bony ring joined to the spine at the sacrum and to the legs at the hip joints
perception - a person's knowledge of the physical world as interpreted by the brain
perianal - surrounding the anus
periosteum - outer covering of bone
peripheral - away from the central part of the body, usually referring to structures in the arms and legs
peripheral nervous system - the nerves of the body, peripheral to the spinal cord
perirectal - area surrounding the anus and end part of the rectum
pharmacology - the study of drugs and their effects on the body

physiatrist - an MD specializing in physical medicine and non-surgical rehabilitation

physical therapy - an allied health profession which uses physical means to promote health and rehabilitation

pia mater - the innermost of the three meninges

piriformis - a muscle in the buttock through or under which the sciatic nerve passes

piriformis syndrome - a condition in which spasm of the piriformis muscle causes sciatic nerve compression

placebo - treatment which has no beneficial physical effects

placebo effect - relief of symptoms following the use of a placebo

posterior - toward the back of the body

posterior superior iliac spine - bony landmark on the pelvis near the top of the sacrum

posterolateral - angled toward the back and side of the body

post-op - following a surgical procedure

posture - the position one assumes against gravity

pre-op - preceding a surgical procedure

press-ups - an exercise of passive hyperextension in prone, used for disk prolapse

prognosis - outlook of an illness; chances for recovery

prolapsed disk - condition in which the nucleus of the disk pushes against the annular fibers, causing them to bulge into the spinal canal

proliferant - substance which stimulates the production of new tissue

prone - stomach-lying

protrusion - bulging of tissue beyond its normal boundary

PSIS - posterior superior iliac spine

psychiatrist - an MD specializing in treatment of emotional or mental problems

psychogenic - originating in the mind

PT - physical therapy or physical therapist

pubic symphysis - fibrous joint at the front of the pelvis

pubis - anterior part of the pelvis

pyriformis - see piriformis

Qi - Chinese concept meaning the body's vital energy

radiation - movement of symptoms from an injured area, often following the path of a nerve; electromagnetic waves

radicular - pertaining to a specific nerve root and its distribution

radiographic - pertaining to diagnostic tests in which x-rays or other electromagnetic waves are used to visualize internal parts of the body, including x-rays, CAT scans, MRI, myelograms, bone scans, etc.

radiologic/radiological - see radiographic

radiologist - an MD specializing in the performance and interpretation of radiographic testing

range of motion - the full arc of movement available at a joint

reciprocal inhibition - technique using a strong contraction of a tight muscle which causes subsequent inhibition and relaxation of that muscle

rectal tone - responsiveness of the sphincter muscles responsible for bowel retention

rectus - the abdominal muscle which performs straight trunk flexion

reflex - an immediate motor response following a sensory stimulus which initially bypasses the brain

reflex inhibition - reduction of muscle spasm through the use of nervous system mechanisms

residency - hospital training for MDs or DOs following internship, for specialization rheumatoid - pertaining to the joints of the body

ROM - see range of motion

rotation - twisting movement around a body axis

ruptured disk - a condition in which part of the nucleus of a disk has extruded through the outer annular fibers into the spinal canal

sacro-iliac joint - the connection between the pelvis and sacrum

sacro-iliac joint dysfunction - a syndrome in which the SI joint is subluxed, inflamed or painful

sacral - pertaining to the spinal region between the low back and tailbone

sacrum - five vertebrae located below the lumbar vertebrae which are fused into one bone

sciatica - pain which follows the path of the sciatic nerve down the back of the leg

sciatic nerve - large nerve composed of a bundle of nerve fibers from the lumbar and sacral parts of the spinal cord, which runs down the back of the thigh and innervates the posterior thigh, lower leg and foot

sclerotome - deep tissues which are innervated by the one spinal nerve

scoliosis - lateral curvature of the spine

secondary gains - benefits resulting from an illness

sensory stimulation - any input that sends messages about touch, temperature, vibration, movement, etc. through the sensory receptors to the central nervous system

sequestration - condition in which a fragment from the nucleus of a disk is loose in the spinal canal

sheath - outer covering of a nerve or muscle

SI - sacro-iliac

SIJ - sacro-iliac joint

SIJD - sacro-iliac joint dysfunction

SLR - straight leg raise

somatic - pertaining to the body

somatic dysfunction - term used in osteopathy to indicate a functional disorder of the musculo-skeletal system

somatogenic - originating in the body

spasm - painful sustained contraction of a muscle in response to an injury to the muscle or to other nearby structures

specialist - an MD or DO who has completed a residency program in a specialty field

sphincter - muscle which allows retentive control of the bladder or bowel

spinal canal - the space within the vertebral column in which the spinal cord is located

spinal column - vertebral column; the bony spine

spinal cord - structure containing bundles of nerves which connects the brain and peripheral nervous system and which is enclosed by the spinal column

spinal muscles - four muscles composed of short fibers which originate and insert on the vertebrae and which extend and stabilize the spine

spinous process - posterior bony projection of a vertebra

spondylolysis - defect in the bony arch of a vertebra causing spinal instability

spondylolisthesis - bilateral defect of the bony arch of a vertebra with anterior slipping of the affected vertebral body

spondylosis - degenerative disease of the spine, with changes of vertebrae, joints and disks

sprain - injury or tearing of ligaments

stenosis - abnormal congenital or degenerative narrowing of the spinal canal

straight leg raise - a test for nerve root compression in which the hip is flexed with the knee extended; an exercise to stretch the hamstring muscle

straights - chiropractors who limit their practice to manipulation of the spinal column

strain - injury or tearing of muscle tissue

strain-counterstrain - a technique using passive positioning to reduce sensory input from soft tissues in order to reduce muscle tone

strength - the amount of resistance a muscle can overcome in a single repetition

structure - physical components of the body

subchondral bone - part of a bone located below the articular cartilage

subluxation - partial disruption of the opposing surfaces of a joint; slight vertebral malalignment

supine - back-lying

sympathetic nervous system - throacolumbar portion of the autonomic nervous system

symptom - a change in a patient's condition, indicating a dysfunctional state

syndrome - a set of symptoms which occur together, indicating a specific medical condition

synovial fluid - substance produced by the lining of a joint to provide shock-absorption, lubrication and protection for the joint

synovial joint - joint surrounded by a fluid-producing synovial membrane; a joint with a measurable amount of movement

synovial lining/membrane - the inner lining of a joint which secretes synovial fluid

systemic - affecting the whole body

tendon - non-elastic part of a muscle; inelastic cord which attaches a muscle to a bone

tendonitis - inflammation of a tendon

tenosynovitis - inflammation of a tendon and synovial membrane of a joint

TENS - see transcutaneous electrical nerve stimulation

therapeutic - beneficial; causing reversal of pathology or symptoms

thermograph - diagnostic tool which measures spinal heat

thoracic - pertaining to the trunk or to the part of the spine between the neck and waist

thrust - a sudden, high-velocity, low amplitude force applied to a specific structure of the body

tone - readiness of a muscle to contract; a muscle's resistance to stretch

total bedrest - see bedrest

toxic - poisonous to the body

traction - a pulling force which separates joint surfaces

transcutaneous electrical nerve stimulation - a modality which imparts a mild electrical current to the skin to inhibit pain elsewhere in the body

transverse ligaments - short ligaments connecting the transverse processes of two vertebrae

transverse process - bony lateral projection of a vertebra to which muscles and ligaments attach

trigger point - most tender spot in a muscle; tender area of fibrous bands in a muscle

trochanter - bony prominence on the femur

trochanteric belt - stabilizing support which surrounds the pelvis at hip level to provide support for the SI joint

tropism - degenerative scoliosis of individual spinal segments caused by asymmetry of disks or vertebrae

ultra-sound - machine which uses sound waves to produce heat in deep tissues

Valsalva maneuver - tightening of the abdominal muscles with a closed glottis; straining

vascular - having a large blood supply

vertebra - single bony segment of the spinal column

vertebrae - plural of vertebra

vertebral body - the largest part of a vertebra, separated from other vertebral bodies by disks vertebral column - spinal column; bony spine

vertebral process - one of a number of bony projections of a vertebra

viscera - the large interior organs of the body

Williams flexion exercises - a treatment regime for low back pain which emphasizes flexion postures and abdominal strengthening

work hardening - a treatment program which simulates a patient's work environment in order to return injured workers to the job safely and quickly

x-ray - a radiographic test in which the bones of the body are visualized

yin and yang - names for the Chinese concept of the two opposing influences on the body

Appendix B

Chronic Back Pain Survey

This survey will be used for a study comparing the various approaches which are used in the treatment of chronic back pain, (pain of six months duration or more).

Was onset of pain sudden, gradual or intermittent? What were the circumstances?

_____

_____

_____

Duration of pain in months/years. Area and description of pain:

_____

_____

Please list the treatments tried, the health care provider supervising the treatments and the results (pro or con).

1)

2)

3)

4)

What has been the most difficult aspect for you of having chronic pain?

_____

_____

What has helped you to cope with the pain from a physical standpoint? from an emotional standpoint?

_____

_____

_____

Further comments:

_____

_____

_____

Name:_____

Address: _____

Phone: _____

The following results are based on the above survey which was distributed to people with chronic back pain. The size of the sample is too small to be statistically significant, but the results support the author's view – no one treatment for back pain helps every patient. Klein & Sobel's book, *Backache Relief*, reports the results of an extensive survey of back patients; they reach the same conclusion.

Treatment/Prof.	Very Helpful	Somewhat Helpful	Not Helpful/ Made Worse
acupuncture	2	2	0
anti-inflammatories	0	0	4
back exercises	5	0	0
bedrest	0	4	3
body mechanics	3	1	0
braces	1	2	0
biofeedback	0	1	0
chiropractor	1	1	6
cold	0	1	1
counseling	0	1	0
foot reflexology	1	0	0
heat	0	2	1
injection	0	1	2
marijuana	0	1	0
massage	0	0	1
meditation	2	0	0
mind over back pain	1	0	0
muscle relaxants	0	2	1
orthopedist	0	1	1
osteopath	1	5	6
pain killers	0	5	4
phys. conditioning	1	0	0
physical therapy	1	3	8
surgery	3	2	2
TENS	1	0	1
traction	0	0	1

Appendix C

Bibliography

Abraham, Edward, *Freedom from Back Pain: An Orthopedist's Self-Help Guide*, Rodale, 1986

Allen, Henry, "That Back's Gotta Come Out," *The Washington Post*, April 29, 1990

American Medical Association, *The American Medical Association Book of Back Care*, Random House, 1982

American Osteopathic Association, informational literature, 1987-1989

"Approaches to Musculoskeletal Problems: Focus on the Low Back," Robert M. True, M.D. Symposium, April 26-27, 1985, South Portland, Maine

Apts, David & Blankenship, Keith, *Back Facts for the American Back School*, FPR, Inc., 1981

The Back Letter, "Memo on Body Mechanics," Ed. Theresa Reger, Skol Publishing

The Back Letter, Ed. Theresa Reger, Skol Publishing, Vol. 4, No. 2-9, December 1989-July, 1990

Barnes, John, "Benefits of Myofascial Release, Craniosacral Therapy Explained," *Physical Therapy Forum*, Aug., 29, 1984

Barnes, John, "Pro: Never Trademarked Myofascial Release," *P.T. Bulletin*, Feb. 17, 1988

Barnes, John, "Therapeutic Insight," *Physical Therapy Forum*, June 25, 1986

Batson, Glenna, "Reeducating or Strengthening: Relooking at the Pelvic Tilt," *Physical Therapy Forum*, Oct. 2, 1985

Beal, Myron, "The Sacroiliac Problem: Review of Anatomy, Mechanics and Diagnosis," *Journal of Amer. Osteopathic Assoc.*, Vol. 81, No. 10, June, 1982

Bellamy, Nicholas, Park, William & Rooney, Patrick, "What Do We Know About the Sacroiliac Joint," *Seminars in Arthritis and Rheumatism*, Vol. 12, No. 3, February, 1983

Benanti, Joseph & Ellis, Jeffrey, "Holistic Medicine a 'Crisis' for PTs," *PT Bulletin*, Jan. 18, 1989

Benjamin, Ben, "The Mystery of Lower Back Pain," Parts I & II, *Massage Therapy Journal*, Fall 1988 & Winter 1989

Blackburn, Stan & Portney, Leslie Gross, "Electromyographic Activity of Back Musculature During Williams' Flexion Exercises," Physical Therapy, Vol. 61, No. 6, June, 1981

Brena, Steven F., *Chronic Pain: America's Hidden Epidemic*, Atheneum/SMI, 1978

Bunch, Richard, "Con: Myofascial Release Traced Back Decades," *P.T. Bulletin*, Feb. 17, 1988

Burkart, Sandy & Beresford, William, "The Aging Intervertebral Disk," *Physical Therapy*, Vol. 59, No. 8, August, 1979

Cailliet, Rene, *Low Back Pain Syndrome*, Second Edition, F.A. Davis, 1962

Cailliet, Rene, *Low Back Pain Syndrome*, Edition 4, F.A. Davis, 1988

Caplan, Deborah, *Back Trouble*, Triad Publishing Co., 1987

Carmichael, Joel, "Inter- and Intra-Examiner Reliability of Palpation for Sacroiliac Joint Dysfunction," *Journal of Manipulative and Physiological Therapeutics*, Vol. 10, No. 4, August, 1987

Carper, Jean, *Health Care U.S.A.*, Prentice Hall Press, 1987

Carr, Sharon & Phillips, Cathy L., "Helping TMJ Patients to Help Themselves," *Physical Therapy Forum*, Jan. 8, 1990

101

Carroll, Sarah, "Hypnosis: An Underutilized Modality," *Physical Therapy Forum*

Carter, Mildred, *Helping Yourself With Foot Reflexology*, Parker Publishing Co., 1969

Cassel, Eric, "The Nature of Suffering and the Goals of Medicine," *New England Journal of Medicine*, Vol. 306, No. 11, March 18, 1982

Chapman-Smith, David, "Chiropractic – A Referenced Source of Modern Concepts, New Evidence," Practice Makers Products Inc., 1988

CIBA Clinical Symposia,"Low Back Pain," Vol. 25, Number 3, CIBA Pharmaceutical Co., 1973

Cibulka, Michael & Koldehoff, Rhonda, "Evaluating Chronic Sacroiliac Joint Dysfunction," *Clinical Management*, Vol. 6, No. 4, 1987

Cibulka, Michael & Koldehoff, Rhonda, "Leg Length Disparity and Its Effect on Sacroiliac Joint Dysfunction," *Clinical Management*, Vol. 6, No. 5, 1987

Colbin, Annemarie, *Food and Healing*, Ballantine Books, 1986

Consumer Reports Books, Editors of, *Health Quackery: Consumers Union's Report on False Health Claims, Worthless Remedies and Unproved Therapies, Holt, Rhinehart and Winston, 1980*

Cousins, Norman, *Anatomy of an Illness*, W.W. Norton & Co., 1979

Croce, Pat, "Put Stress to Rest," *Physical Therapy Forum*, August 21, 1989

Cuckler, John, Bernini, Philip, Wiesel, Sam, Booth, Robert, Ruthman, Richard & Pickens, Gary, "The Use of Epidural Steroids in the Treatment of Lumbar Radicular Pain," The Journal of Bone & Joint Surgery, Vol. 67-A, No. 1, January, 1985

Cyriax, James, *Textbook of Orthopaedic Medicine*, Baillier-Tindall, 1980

Derebery, Jane & Tullis, William, "Delayed Recovery in the Patient with a Work Compensable Injury," *Journal of Occupational Medicine*, Nov., 1983

Deyo, Richard, "Conservative Therapy for Low Back Pain," *JAMA*, Aug. 26, 1983, Vol. 250

Deyo, Richard, Loeser, John & Bigos, Stanley, "Herniated Lumbar Intervertebral Disk," *Annals of Internal Medicine*, Vol. 112, No. 8, April 15, 1990

Deyo, Richard, Walsh, Nicholas, Martin, Donald, Schoenfeld, Lawrence & Ramamurthy, Somayaji, "A Controlled Trial of Transcutaneous Electrical Nerve Stimulation (TENS) and Exercise for Chronic Low Back Pain," *The New England Journal of Medicine*, Vol. 322, No. 23, June 7, 1990

DiFabio, Richard, "Clinical Assessment of Manipulation and Mobilization of the Lumbar Spine," *Physical Therapy*, Vol. 66, No. 1, Jan., 1986

Dimick, Terry, "Kinesiotherapist Responds," *P.T. Bulletin*, July 4, 1990

Dommerholt, Jan, "Meridian Therapy – A New European Concept," *Physical Therapy Forum*, March 5, 1990

DonTigny, Richard, "Dysfunction of the Sacroiliac Joint and Its Treatment," *The Journal of Orthopaedic and Sports Medicine Therapy*, Vol. 1, No. 1, Summer, 1979

DonTingy, Richard, "Function and Pathomechanics of the Sacroiliac Joint," *Physical Therapy*, Vol. 65, No. 1, Jan., 1985

Edgelow, Peter, "Physical Examination of the Lumbosacral Complex," *Physical Therapy*, Vol. 59, No. 8, Aug., 1979

Elgee, Neil, "Norman Cousins' Sick Laughter Redux," *Archives of Internal Medicine*, Vol. 150, August, 1990

Fager, Charles, "Beware the Quick Fix for Back Pain," *Trends in Rehabilitation*, Winter, 1986

Fager, Charles, "Facts and Fallacies of Spinal Disorders: A Neurosurgeon's Viewpoint," *Evaluation and Treatment of Chronic Pain*

Fager, Charles, "The Neurosurgical Management of Lumbar Spine Disease," *New Developments in Medicine*, Vol. 3, No. 2, Sept., 1988
Fahey, Brian, "The Principles of Structural Diagnosis," *Physical Therapy Forum*, Oct. 23, 1989
Folan, Lilias, *Lilias Yoga and You*, Bantum Books,1972
Friedman, Nancy, "Back Exercises for a Healthy Back," Krames Communications, 1985

Gildenberg, Philip L. & DeVaul, Richard A., *The Chronic Pain Patient*, Kargen, 1985
Glade, Phyllis, *Crystal Healing: The Next Step*, Llewellyn Publications, 1989
Glisan, Billy, Stith, William & Kiser, Sanford, "Physiology of Active Exercise in Rehabilitation of Back Injuries," *Health Tracks*, Vol. 2, Issue 1
Goering, Gail, "Treat Injured Workers Like Athletes," *P.T. Bulletin*, May 9, 1990
Gottlieb, Harold, Alperson, Burton, Koller, Reuben & Hockersmith, Virgil, "An Innovative Program for the Restoration of Patients with Chronic Back Pain," *Physical Therapy*, Vol. 59, No. 8, August, 1979
Grieve, Elizabeth "Lumbo-pelvic Rhythm and Mechanical Dysfunction of the Sacro-iliac Joint," *Physiotherapy*, Vol. 67, No. 6, June, 1981

Hay, Louise, *You Can Heal Your Life*, Hay House, 1984
Headley, Barbara, *Chronic Pain: Life Out of Balance*, H. Duane Saunders, 1987
Headley, Barbara, "Dynamic Stabilization," *Physical Therapy Forum*, June 4, 1990
Headley, Barbara, "Pain Vs. Suffering," *Physical Therapy Forum*, May 16, 1988
Headley, Barbara, "Postural Homeostasis," *Physical Therapy Forum*, Sept. 17, 1990
Hebert, Lauren, *Sex and Back Pain*, H. Duane Saunders, 1987
Heinrich, Steve, "Body Watch: The Importance of Dialogue and Myofascial Unwinding in Creating a Safe Place to Heal," *Physical Therapy Forum*, Feb. 5, 1990
Heller, Joseph & Hanson, Jan, *The Client's Handbook*, The Body of Knowledge, Mt. Shasta, Ca.
Horwich, Mark, "Low Back Pain: The Neurologist's View," *Drug Therapy*, Dec., 1982
Hutchinson, Lynn, "Direct Access and Preventative Therapy," *Physical Therapy Forum*, Sept., 25, 1989

Imrie, David, *Goodbye Back Ache*, Prentice-Hall/Newcastle, 1983
Irwin, Yukiko, *Shiatzu*, J.B. Lippincott, 1976
Ishmael, William & Shorbe, Howard, "Care of the Back," J.B. Lippincott Co., 1953

Jackson, Claudia & Brown, Mark, "Analysis of Current Approaches and a Practical Guide to Prescription of Exercise," *Clinical Orthopaedics*, No. 179, October, 1983
Jackson, Claudia & Brown, Mark, "Is There a Role for Exercise in the Treatments of Patients with Low Back Pain", *Clinical Orthopaedics*, No. 179, October 1983
Jacobs, Bernard, "Low Back Pain: The Orthopedist's View," *Drug Therapy*, Dec., 1982
Jones, Bob, *The Difference a D.O. Makes*, Osteopathic Medicine in the Twentieth Century, Times-Journal Publishing Co., Oklahoma City, Ok., 1978
Jones, Frank Pierce, *Body Awareness in Action: A Study of the Alexander Technique*, Schocken Books, 1979

Kaplan, Paul & Tanner, Ellen, *Musculoskeletal Pain and Disability*, Appleton & Lange, 1989
Kessler, Randolph, "Acute Symptomatic Disk Prolapse," *Physical Therapy*, Vol. 59, No. 8, Aug., 1979

Kessler, Randolph & Hertling, Darlene, *Management of Common Musculoskeletal Disorders*, Harper & Row, 1983

Kim, Nini, "Holistic Medicine Requires Different World View," *PT Bulletin*, March 1, 1989

Kirkaldy-Willis, W.H., *Managing Low Back Pain*, Churchill Livingstone, 1988

Kirkaldy-Willis, W.H. & Hill, R.J., "A More Precise Diagnosis for Low Back Pain," *Spine* Vol. 4, No. 2, Mar./Apr., 1979

Klein, Arthur & Sobel, Dava, *Backache Relief*, New American Library, 1985

Knott, Margaret & Voss, Dorothy, *Proprioceptive Neuramuscular Facilitation*, Harper & Row, 1968

Kotzsch, Ronald, "AIDS: Putting an Alternative to the Test," *East West*, Sept., 1986

Krumhansl, Bernice & Nowacek, Charles, "Case Study – Spinal Manipulation Under Anaesthesia," *Physical Therapy Forum*, Sept. 4, 1989

Lamb, David, "The Neurology of Spinal Pain," *Physical Therapy*, Vol. 59, No. 8, Aug., 1979

Langone, John, *Chiropractors: A Consumer's Guide*, Addison-Wesley Publiching Co., 1982

Lauterback, Joyce, "The Mind-Body Connection – Is There More?" *Physical Therapy Forum*, July 17, 1989

Lawn, George, "How to Lift – Is There a Right Way?" *Physical Therapy Forum*, June 12, 1985

Lehman, Betsy, "Feeling Bad About Feeling Bad," *The Good Health Magazine (Boston Globe)*, October 8, 1989

Levine, David B., *The Painful Low Back*, Merck, Sharp & Dohme, 1979

Lewith, Geroge & Horn, Sandra, *Drug Free Pain Relief*, Thorsons Publishers, 1987

Lockett, Ricky, "Pyriformis Syndrome – Diagnosis and Treatment," *Physical Therapy Forum*, Aug. 22, 1988

MacPhee, Patricia, "Chronic Pain and the Role of Occupational Therapy," *Physical Therapy Forum*, Sept. 18, 1989

Maitland, G.D., *Vertebral Manipulation*, Butterworths, 1977

Marantz, Steve, "The Perfect Chair," *The Boston Globe*, Oct. 8, 1989

Mayer, Tom, "Rehabilitation of the Patient with Spinal Pain," *The Orthopedic Clinics of North America*, Vol. 14, No. 3, July 1983

McGavin, James, "The McKenzie Approach to Spinal Pain," *Physical Therapy Forum*, July 5, 1988

McKenzie, Robin, *Treat Your Own Back*, Spinal Publications Ltd., 1985

McGregor, Marion & Cassidy, David, "Post-surgical Sacroiliac Joint Syndrome," *Journal of Manipulative and Physiologic Therapeutics*, Vol. 6, No. 1, March, 1983

Mead, Mark, "Chiropractic's New Wave," *East West*, November, 1989

Melnick, Michael, Saunders, Robin & Saunders, Duane, *Managing Back Pain*, H. Duane Saunders, 1989

Miller, David, "Comparison of Electromyographic Activity in the Lumbar Paraspinal Muscles of Subjects with and without Low Back Pain," *Physical Therapy*, Vol. 65, No. 9, Sept., 1985

Mills, Simon & Finando, Steven, *Alternatives in Healing: An Open-Minded Approach to Finding the Best Treatment for Your Health Problems*, New American Library, 1989

Mixter, Jason, "Rolfing," (Editors) Lowe & Nechas, *Whole Body Healing*, Rodale Press, 1983

Montgomery, Edith, "Folsom Physical Therapy – A Different Approach to Back Rehabilitation," *Physical Therapy Forum*, June 13, 1988

Olsen, Paulette, "Body Mechanics Education – A Legacy for our Children," *Physical Therapy Forum*, April 23, 1990

Olsen, Paulette, "Brief Media Presentations on Back Care," *Physical Therapy Forum*, Nov. 27, 1989

Ondricek, Jana, "Techniques for Effective Therapeutic Management of Workmen's Compensation Patients," *Physical Therapy Forum*, April 30, 1990

Ongley, Milne, Klein, Robert, Dorman, Thomas, Eek, Bjorn, & Hubert, Lawrence, "A New Approach to the Treatment of Chronic Back Pain," *The Lancet*, July 18, 1987

Paris, Stanley, "Anatormy as Related to Function and Pain," *The Orthopedic Clinics of North America*, Vol. 14, No. 3, July, 1983

Paris, Stanley, "Mobilization of the Spine," *Physical Therapy*, Vol. 59, No. 8, Aug., 1979

Paris, Stanley, "Physical Signs of Instability," *Spine*, Vol. 10, No. 3, 1985

Paris, Stanley, *The Spine*, (Course Notes), Stanley Paris, 1979

Picker, Robert, "Microcurrent Therapy: 'Jump-Starting' Healing with Bioelectricity," *Physical Therapy Forum*, June 10, 1989

Pitzele, Sefra Korbin, *We Are Not Alone: Learning to Live with Chronic Illness*, Workman Publishing, 1985

Potter, Nancy & Rothstein, Jules, "Intertester Reliability for Selected Clinical Tests of the Sacroiliac Joint," *Physical Therapy*, Vol. 65, No. 11, Nov., 1985

Prudden, Bonnie, *Pain Erasure*, Ballantine Books, 1980

P.T. Bulletin, "Benefits of 'Humor Therapy' Promoted," April 25, 1980

P.T. Bulletin, "Reactions Mixed to Back Surgery Alternative," August 30, 1989

Rashbaum, Ralph, "Radiofrequency Facet Denervation," *The Orthopedic Clinics of North America*, Vol. 14, No. 3, July, 1983

Reese, David, "Keep PT the Art That It Is," *P.T. Bulletin*, April 25, 1990

Register, Cheri, *Living with Chronic Illness: Days of Patience and Passion*, The Free Press (Maacmillan), 1987

Reuben, Carolyn, "AIDS: The Promise of Alternative Treatments," *East West*, Sept., 1986

Rice, John, Allen, Nancy & Caldwell, David, "Low Back Pain: The Rheumatologist's View," *Drug Therapy*, Dec., 1982

Richardson, Nancy, "Aston-Patterning," *Physical Therapy Forum*, Oct., 28, 1987

Rolf, Ida, "Structural Integration," *Confin. Psychiat.* 16, 1973

Sarno, John, *Mind Over Back Pain*, Berkley Books, 1982

Saunders, H. Duane, *The Back Care Program*, H. Duane Saunders, 1983

Saunders, H. Duane, *Evaluation, Treatment and Prevention of Musculoskeletal Disorders*, H. Duane Saunders, 1985

Saunders, Duane, *For Your Neck*, H. Duane Saunders, 1986

Shapiro, Gary, "Ceasing the Struggle," *Physical Therapy Forum*, May 7, 1990

Shea, Michael, "MFR and the Psychosomatio Body," *Physical Therapy Forum*, April 23, 1990

Sherman, Carl, "The Medicolegal Thicket of Low Back Disability," *Aches and Pains*, April, 1982

Siegel, Bernie S., *Peace, Love and Healing*, Harper & Row, 1989

Simons, David & Travell, Janet, "Myofascial Origins of Low Back Pain," Parts 1-3, *Postgraduate Medicine*, Vol. 73, No. 2, Feb., 1983

Smith, Ralph Lee, *At Your Own Risk: The Case Against Chiropractic*, Trident Press, 1969

Solet, Jo, "Low Back Pain – An Overview," *Physical Therapy Forum*, August 7, 1989

Steer, Allen, Hardin, John & Malawista, Stephen, "Lyme Arthritis: A New Clinical Entity," *Hospital Practice*, April, 1978

Sternbach, Richard A., *Pain Patients; Traits and Treatments*, Academic Press, 1974

Stickland, Ellen, "Trouble with KTs," *PT Bulletin*

Tamayo, Rey, "Work Hardening – A Different Treatment Approach," *Physical Therapy Forum*, Feb. 26, 1990

Thomas, Lynn, Hislop, Helen & Waters, Robert, "Physiological Work Performance in Chronic Low Back Disability," *Physical Therapy*, Vol. 60, No. 4, April, 1980

Wallnofer, Heinrich & vonRottauscher, Anna, *Chinese Folk Medicine and Acupuncture*, Bell Publishing Co., 1965

Weiselfish, Sharon & Kain, Jay, "Introduction of Developmental Manual Therapy – An Integrated System Approach for Structural and Functional Rehabilitation," *Physical Therapy Forum*, Feb. 12, 1990

White, Arthur, "Injection Techniques for the Diagnosis and Treatment of Low Back Pain," *The Orthopedic Clinics of North America*, Vol. 14, No. 3, July, 1983

Wildman, Frank, "The Feldenkrais Method: Clinical Applications," *P.T. Forum*, Feb. 19, 1986

Wildman, Frank, "Learning – The Missing Link in Physical Therapy," *P.T. Forum*, Feb. 8, 1988

Wildman, Frank, "Training in the Feldenkrais Method," The Institute for Movement Studies, Berkeley, Ca.

Wilk, Chester, *Chiropractic Speaks Out*, Wilk Publishing Co., 1973

Willis, Judith, "Back Pain: Ubiquitous, Controversial," *FDA Consumer*, November, 1983

Wolf, Barbara, *Living With Pain*, The Seabury Press, 1977

Woodworth, Barbara, "Therapeutic Values of Tai Chi," *Physical Therapy Forum*, July 23, 1990

Wyatt, William, DO, literature for patients, 1987

Yunus, Muhammed, Masi, Alfonse, Calabro, John & Shah, Indravadan, "Primary Fibromyalgia," *Amer. Fam. Phys.*, May, 1982

Zacharkow, Dennis, "The Problems with Lumbar Support," *Physical Therapy Forum*, Sept. 10, 1990

Zimmerman, Julie, *Goals and Objectives for Developing Normal Movement Patterns*, Aspen, 1988

Zinman, David, "Focus on Back Pain," *Newsday*, Jan. 30, 1990

Index - Chronic Back Pain: Moving On

family/friends 10, 39-40, 43-4, 47-50, 78-9, 82-5
fascia 22, 23-4, 33
fatigue 44
feelings (see attitude; emotional/psych. factors)
financial compensation 6, 41; f. cost of back pain 6
flexibility (see exercises; range of motion)
flexion 23
frustration (see emotional/psych. factors)

gate control theory 31, 55-6
guilt (see emotional/psych. factors)

heat 74
hip joint [Fig. 1-2]
holism 58
home programs 71-5
housekeeping 79-80
humor 55, 84
hypnosis 64, 67-8

ice 74-5
ilium (pl. ilia) 16 [Fig. 1-2]
independence with chronic pain 78-81, 84
individualization of treatment 9-11, 41, 54, 59, 65, 71, 74, 82
inflammation 23, 57-8, 74-5
inhibition (see muscle i.; pain i.)
injections 59-60
instability (see facet joint dysfunction, sacro-iliac joint dysfunc.)
intervertebral disks (see disks)
ischium 16 [Fig. 1-2]
isolation (see emotional effects of pain; e. influences on pain)

job injuries (see work injuries; worker's compensation)
jogging (see running)
joint capsule 16, 22 [Fig. 1-8C]
joint dysfunction (see facet jnt. dysf., SIJ dysf.)
joint play 23
joints 16, 22-3 [Fig. 1-8]

kyphosis 15

laughter (see humor)
leisure activities 46
lifestyle changes 10, 65-6, 78
lifting (see posture/body mechanics)
ligaments 16; sprain 23 (see soft tissues)
locked back (see facet joint dysfunction)
longitudinal ligaments 16, 30 [Fig. 1-5, 1-7]
lordosis 15 (see spinal curves)

low back syndrome 6, 9, 23
lumbar spine 15 [Fig. 1-1]
lying down 72, 80-1

malingering 36, 40
management (see pain coping)
manipulation 54
manual therapy (see manipulation; mobilization)
massage 67
mechanical supports 72
medications 57-8, 64, 72
meditation 67-8
meninges 22
meniscus 16 [Fig. 1-8C]
misdiagnosis 6, 8
mobilization 54
movement 16, 22-3
movement patterns 74
movement reeducation 74
muscles 16, 22-3 [Fig. 1-8]; m. inhibition 67; m. strain/spasm 23-4, 28, 33, 66-7

neck collars 72
negativity (see attitude)
nerve roots 22 [Fig. 1-3]; n.r. compression 23, 28, 59-60 [Fig. 1-10]
nervous system 22
nucleus pulposis (see disks)
nutrition (see diet)

osteopathy (see manipulation)

pain 22, 29-34; p. clinics 63-5; p. coping/management 63-6, 81-2; p. inhibition 53-60; (see chronic pain; perception of pain)
pain-killers (see injections; medications)
pelvic tilts 73-4
pelvis 16 [Fig. 1-2]
perception of pain 29-33, 53, 63, 66
personality and pain (see attitude; emotional/psych. factors)
physical conditioning 54, 67, 73
physical limits (see balance of rest/activity)
piriformis muscle 24, 28 [Fig. 1-13]
piriformis syndrome 24, 28
placebo effect 31-2, 54, 72
positioning 73-4; equipment for p. 72-5
positive attitude (see attitude)
posture/body mechanics 24, 33, 73-4
prevalence of back pain 6
prolapse, disk (see disks)
psychogenic pain 33, 36-41
psychological (see emotional/psych. factors)

The Diagnosis and Misdiagnosis of Back Pain

A complete guide to the causes of bad backs and how professionals diagnose them, by Julie Zimmerman, PT.

Table of Contents

The Almanac of Back Pain Treatments

A complete guide to the rationales, benefits and risks of the traditional and alternative treatments for bad backs, by Julie Zimmerman, PT.

Table of Contents

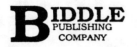

Order Form

Please send

_____ copies of *The Diagnosis and Misdiagnosis of
Back Pain* at $9.95 each $ _____

_____ copies of *The Almanac of Back Pain Treatments*
at $9.95 each $ _____

_____ copies of *Chronic Back Pain: Moving On*
at $9.95 each $ _____

                                                    Subtotal $ _____

For orders of 3-5 books, deduct 15%
For orders of 6 or more books, deduct 20%.   – _____

Sales in state of Maine, add 5% sales tax.   + _____

Shipping, add $1.75 for first book, and $.75 for
each additional book.   + _____

                                        Total enclosed $ _____

Send check payable to: Biddle Publishing Company
                                      Box 1305 - #103
                                      Brunswick, Maine 04011

Expect up to four weeks for delivery.

For inquiries regarding discounts on larger orders, call 207-833-5016.